Praise For Kathryn R. Simpson

"Kathryn Simpson's book is a must-read for anyone with MS, as well as family members and physicians of patients with MS and other neurodegenerative diseases. The merits of this book are immense—it is, to my knowledge, the first book where the major link between neurodegenerative disease and hormone deficiencies and imbalances has been presented. It is essential for a simple reason: It focuses on what actually are, in my experience, the most efficient tools to treat neurodegenerative diseases such as MS—hormone therapies for the endocrine deficiencies that are often associated with these diseases. A major plus for Kathryn Simpson's book is its accurate and easy to understand information on hormone therapies as well as other interventions such as diet improvement and nutritional supplements that boost the efficacy and safety of the hormone therapies."

—Thierry Hertoghe, M.D.
President of the International Hormone Society
President of the World Society of Anti-Aging Medicine
Author of The Hormone Handbook

"I had progressively worsening MS for 10 years before I started on a hormone protocol based on Kathryn Simpson's research. I started on thyroid, estrogen, progesterone and cortisol and my symptoms of chronic fatigue, neuralgia, vision and bladder problems, depression, cognitive dysfunction, tinnitus and breathing difficulty, all resolved very quickly. Anyone who has MS should investigate this treatment—it may be your solution, like it was mine."

—Andrea Jouett
MS Patient

"The amount of information Kathy was able to compile in researching her own MS, and ultimately this book, is truly amazing. Even more amazing were both her rejection of the status quo of current medically recommended therapies and her bravery in trusting her instincts and intellect to take her disease by the horns and resolve all symptoms of her MS by balancing her own hormones—and in the process take control of her health and her life. I've now treated untold numbers of patients with neurodegenerative conditions by testing and treating the hormonal imbalances and deficiencies outlined in this book, and I can attest to the incredible potential this therapy brings."

—Victor W. Rosenfeld, M.D.
Chairman of Neurology and Neurosurgery, Former
Santa Barbara Cottage Hospital

"I was fortunate to have a doctor who implemented Kathryn Simpson's research in his practice. I had suffered with Lupus for over five years, seeing specialist after specialist with symptoms that were getting progressively worse. After going through the testing and evaluation program, it turned out that I had a serious thyroid deficiency as well as a parathyroid disorder. After both were treated, all my symptoms resolved and have been completely gone for over a year now—it's a miracle."

—*Regina Frazier*
Lupus Patient

"Multiple sclerosis is a common disease of unknown cause that strikes relatively young people, especially women, and is currently incurable. This remarkable book offers exciting new insight into MS from researcher—and patient—Kathy Simpson, whose endless energy and commitment is extraordinary. It is a must-read for anyone with MS, anyone who thinks he or she may have MS, and anyone who treats patients with MS."

—*Dale E. Bredesen, M.D.*
Director and CEO
The Buck Institute for Age Research

"After years of treating my patients with traditional therapies, I had the good fortune to meet Kathryn Simpson. After reviewing her extensive research and anecdotal experience, I decided to give hormonal treatment a try with my patients...and the results were amazing. Even long-term cases of MS, fibromyalgia, and lupus responded. Anyone with a neurological disease should have their endocrine function tested to detect deficiencies. All it takes is a simple blood test."

—*William B. Van Valin, II, M.D.*
Chief of Staff, Emeritus
Santa Ynez Valley Cottage Hospital

Other Books by Kathryn R. Simpson

The Perimenopause & Menopause Workbook:
A Comprehensive, Personalized Guide
to Hormonal Health for Women

The Women's Resource Guide to Complete Thyroid Health (2008)

The MS Solution

How I Solved the Puzzle of My Multiple Sclerosis

By Kathryn R. Simpson, M.S.

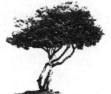

Publisher's Note

The author and publisher have spent considerable time and effort verifying and validating the information included in this book. However, new research is constantly being performed and the information contained herein may become obsolete at any time. As with research, drug protocols are constantly being tested in clinical trials and new drugs are being introduced daily. The dosing levels included are from well-qualified practitioners in the field and are in keeping with current practices at the time of publication, but new drug findings may alter these practices at any time. It is incumbent on every doctor and patient to read labeling data and package inserts thoroughly to make sure that there are no contraindications to use.

Your doctor will be the final judge of what is best in your individual situation, taking into consideration your medical history and current research data. The author is not responsible for any consequences resultant of individual application of the enclosed information, nor for any inadvertent errors or omissions. There is no express or implied warranty in any of the information provided.

Los Olivos Publishing
2720 Ontiveros Rd.
Santa Ynez, CA 93460

Copyright © 2008 by Kathryn R. Simpson.
All rights reserved. No part of this book may be reproduced in any form or by any means, in electronic or mechanical, including photocopying, recording, or by any information storage and retrieval system, without the written permission from publisher.

First Edition
Printed in Thailand

Editor: Jenna Samelson Browning   Proofreader: Jasmine Star
Production: Kimberlee Lynch   Chart Design: Tyler Simpson

Library of Congress Cataloging-in-Publication Data
Simpson, Kathryn R.
    The MS Solution: How I Solved the Puzzle of my Multiple Sclerosis/ Kathryn R. Simpson – 1st ed.
    p. cm.
    ISBN-13: 978-0-9799920-0-1
    ISBN-10: 0-9799920-0-1
Library of Congress Control number: 2007908817

Website: www.hormoneresource.com

To my father, whose courage through progressive neurological disease encouraged me to seek solutions. And to my mother, whose indomitable, pioneer spirit inspired me to fight for my health. And to my husband, Bob, who's had to hear more about hormones than anyone should have to. And to my sons, Tyler, Kyle, and Myles, who have steadfastly stuck by me through illness and the long hours of research my recovery has required.

Acknowledgments

Thanks to Hiram French, Jo Ann Roland, Debbie Merino, Tyler Simpson, Victor Rosenfeld, M.D., Anita Chambers, PhD., William Van Valin II, M.D., and the many doctors, and people with MS, who were willing to take a chance on this unique therapy and share their experiences.

Table of Contents

Authors Note		vi
Foreword		vii
Preface		xi
Chapter I	Finding the MS Solution: My Journey with MS	2
Chapter II	Multiple Sclerosis: An Inflammatory Process	18
Chapter III	Sex Hormones and MS *for Women*	34
Chapter IV	Sex Hormones and MS *for Men*	62
Chapter V	Don't Underestimate Your Thyroid	84
Chapter VI	It's Not Wise to Ignore Your Adrenals	120
Chapter VII	And Let's Not Forget…the Other Hormones	140
Chapter VIII	What Else Does Your Body Need?	154
Final Words	A Message of Hope	182
Appendix A	Recommended Levels	187
Appendix B	Doctor Referrals	190
References		193
Index		201

Author's Note

This book is based on my own personal experience and scientific research. Use it as a starting point in discussing your symptoms, experiences, and treatment with your doctor or other qualified health professional, then together assess whether this information applies to you. Appropriate tests must be conducted so your doctor has a complete picture of your endocrine function. This testing is critical to correctly evaluate your situation and implement the right therapy to address any endocrine imbalances or deficiencies.

This information isn't intended to replace the care of a physician or other licensed health-care professional and shouldn't be taken as medical advice. Do not stop or start treatment without medical oversight—particularly any prescription drugs you are currently taking.

Foreword

Multiple sclerosis is a disease that occurs in approximately 1 out of every 700 people. We've known about it for hundreds of years and it's been studied by tens of thousands of researchers. Billions of dollars have been spent on this research, and yet in the 21st century, when almost anything seems possible, we're left with just a handful of medicines to treat this disease. These drugs are only marginally effective, cost upward of $25,000 a year, and are toxic to the point of causing depression, tissue wasting, and even irreversible, sometimes fatal, brain infections.

How can this be? Part of the problem with current medicine is its uncomfortably close relationship with the pharmaceutical industry. For medical-legal reasons, physicians generally prescribe medicines that have been approved by the FDA. Getting FDA approval is a long, complicated, expensive, and bureaucratic process that for the most part can only be accomplished by the largest pharmaceutical companies willing to gamble tens to hundreds of millions of dollars on developing a product when less than 1 in 300 are approved. Companies have only a few years to recoup the monies spent on developing a drug, gambling also on making large profits before their patent expires and they have to compete with generic versions. Large clinical trials bankrolled by the drug companies and run by physicians who are paid handsomely by these same companies are published in medical journals; the drug companies spend large monies on advertising in these journals, and the products are also reviewed by editors who typically have financial ties to the same companies.

In this climate, it is almost impossible for inexpensive therapies of naturally occurring substances (which are nonpatentable) to be tested in large trials, published in major medical journals, and receive the blessing of the FDA. So we begin to see how some therapies that are inexpensive and potentially very effective may never get formal approval. Yet medicines that cost many thousands of dollars and are potentially fatal do get approved. Physicians are essentially forced into prescribing these therapies because to not do so would be treading on nonapproved, nontested, and potentially litigious ground.

My training and career in neurology has been varied and has included both clinical and bench research, and academic and professional positions. I am currently the department head of a large neurology group in an internationally known multispecialty clinic. This position has afforded me the opportunity to see a large number of patients with a vast array of neurological problems and complaints. One thing that became apparent to me early on is the undeniable relationship between the nervous system and hormones, and also how inadequate my training in medical school was on this subject.

After attending multiple conferences and meetings and reading numerous textbooks on the topic, I now consider myself a *neuroendocrinologist*. The impact this has had on my practice has been life-changing for both my patients and me. Somewhere around 10% of a general neurologists' practice is migraine patients, most are women. In my experience, most of their migraines are related to their menstrual cycle. Wouldn't it behoove all neurologists to take a closer look at this connection? Unfortunately, the vast majority don't ask about hormone issues or test for hormone imbalances, and wouldn't dream of using hormonal therapy to treat these problems. The same can be said for the other conditions we see regularly: epilepsy, sleep disorders, chronic pain, problems associated with head injuries, Parkinson's disease, and of course, multiple sclerosis.

We know that MS is a vastly different process in women than in men. We know that women with MS have worsening symptoms at different points during their menstrual cycle. We know that women who are pregnant have a dramatic reduction in their MS-related exacerbations. It's obvious that hormones are a major factor in MS, and yet how many neurologists do hormonal assessments with their MS patients? I would suspect the number hovers around zero. I've treated untold numbers of patients with neurodegenerative conditions by testing and treating hormonal imbalances and deficiencies, and I can attest to the incredible potential this therapy brings.

Fortunately, at the time of publication there is a major research trial being conducted on at least one hormonal therapy for MS, but clearly more research is needed. However, until the FDA becomes more amenable to inexpensive and practical therapies, and the editors of the medical journals and academic publishers of practice guidelines stop being financially involved with the companies whose products they are supposed to be objectively assessing, hormonal therapies will continue to take a backseat and many patients who could benefit from these therapies will never receive it.

It's a great honor and pleasure for me to write this foreword for Kathy Simpson's book. We have worked together for years and she has given me invaluable input on hormonal treatment of neurological disease. After receiving a diagnosis of MS, Kathy very early on realized that many of her symptoms could also be considered symptoms of hormone deficiency. At a time before Internet search engines could tell you anything you want to know in a matter of seconds, the amount of information she was able to compile on her own in researching her MS, and ultimately this book, is truly amazing. Even more amazing were both her rejection of the status quo of current medically recommended therapies and her bravery in trusting her instincts and intellect to take her disease by the horns and resolve all symptoms of her MS by balancing her own hormones—and in the process take control of her disease and her life. As to not spoil the reading of this book, I will turn you over to Kathy and let her tell you her story, and hopefully open your eyes to the possibilities of what hormonal therapy can offer those who suffer from MS.

—*Victor W. Rosenfeld, M.D.*

Preface

Although it took years of research, I found the solution to my multiple sclerosis symptoms and identified the all-important link between MS and the endocrine system. It's now my goal to share this research with others so that they, too, may find the same relief.

I've explored all avenues to get this information out. I wrote *The Perimenopause & Menopause Workbook* (New Harbinger Publications, 2006), with coauthor Dale Bredesen, M.D., to give women the tools to evaluate their hormone health. As of this writing, I am authoring another book for New Harbinger, this time on thyroid function: *The Women's Resource Guide to Complete Thyroid Health* (2008). I've met with countless doctors to share my science and experience. I opened a clinic with a doctor friend to research and treat hormone imbalances and deficiencies as well as neurodegenerative disease. I'm working with an oncologist friend to launch a clinical study to test the safety and efficacy of bio-identical estrogen and progesterone in treating symptoms of hormone imbalance. I've worked with celebrities to resolve their symptoms (with great success) in the hope that they would help me get the word out. I have talked to numerous groups to raise awareness of the importance of hormones in aging and disease. I'm actively trying to make others who suffer from neurodegenerative disorders—whether MS, PSP (progressive supranuclear palsy), Parkinson's, or others—aware of the role their endocrine system plays in their disease.

This book concentrates all these efforts into one resource, which I hope will give you the tools you need to start the process of evaluating your own situation. My wish is that this truly miraculous therapy will restore your health, and that you will use your newfound energy and renewed lease on life to spread the word to others still suffering from the disease. Good luck and let me know how you do!

—Kathryn R. Simpson, M.S.
info@hormoneresource.com

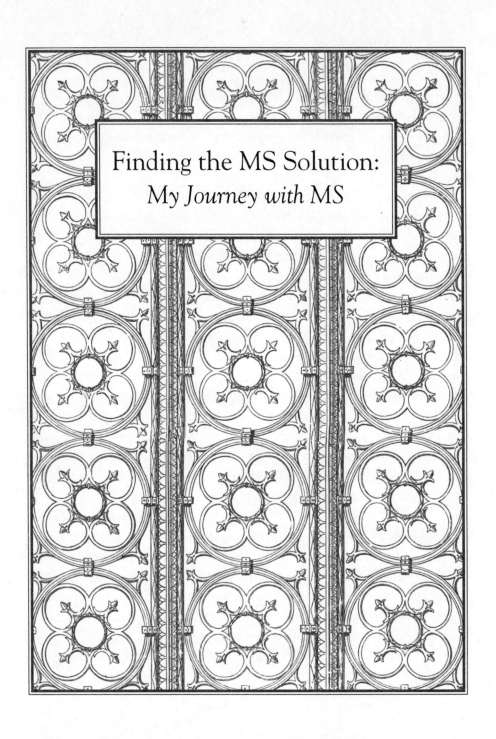

Finding the MS Solution:
My Journey with MS

I

How It All Started

Life was great. I had a good job, a nice husband, and two wonderful sons, had managed to stay slim and trim into my late 30s, and as far as I was concerned, my health was fine. Sure, I had a hard time getting pregnant with my second son and had to undergo fertility treatments, had chronic constipation and sinus infections as far back as I could remember, and sometimes couldn't get to sleep, but I felt great day to day—which, let's face it, is all you really worry about when you're in your 20s and 30s.

Then, six months after the birth of my second son, at 39, my hands began to get numb. It started in my right hand and spread to my left a couple of months later. I went to a neurologist who did a nerve conduction test and told me I had carpal tunnel syndrome and that the only way to resolve it was hand surgery. Not overly inclined to jump into surgery, I decided to look into other options. I went to another doctor who told me that high levels of heavy metals or vitamin and mineral deficiencies also caused peripheral neuropathy (numb hands). Tests showed that I had both—very high levels of mercury and cadmium and low levels of B vitamins—so the doctor started me on a drug to remove the toxic metals from my body and also on vitamin and mineral supplements. After six months, my levels of mercury, cadmium, and B vitamins had returned to normal ranges but the numbness hadn't changed. I didn't have any pain, so I figured I would just wait and see if it got worse. I could always have surgery later.

About this time I took a job as CEO of a start-up company and got so busy I didn't have a minute to think about the numbness. Over the next three years my hands got progressively worse, making it hard to write and pick up small objects, but I was so occupied with work and having my third son that I didn't have much time to do anything about it.

> *I don't have to tell you how insidious this path is. I am willing to bet most of you reading this book have similar stories. We just keep going to one doctor after another with our lists of symptoms. We get one prescription after another and a referral to yet another specialist from our doctors, whose expressions say "hypochondriac," or worse…"crazy."*

It wasn't until age 44 that I started to get other worrisome symptoms. The first thing I noticed was fatigue. I had never had a tired day in my life; I was up and off to work by 7 a.m. every morning and rarely home before 6:30 p.m. Now, it was all I could do to get through the afternoon. Never much of a coffee drinker, I stopped at the corner coffee shop every morning for a double cappuccino on the way to work. This got me through the morning, but then I needed iced tea at lunch and a latte mid-afternoon to get me through the rest of the day. I also found myself getting short-tempered. Always fairly even tempered and not prone to depression or any of the traditional female hormonal challenges like PMS, I couldn't figure out what was going on.

In retrospect, many other gradual changes in my health also occurred during this time. My vision grew much worse and I had to get glasses for computer work and reading. I started to have back problems, with pain and stiffness settling in. I had so much nighttime pain that I woke up throughout the night if I didn't take a sleeping pill. Because I was having a harder and harder time falling asleep anyway, many nights I just gave in and took one. I also felt a sharp pain in my right palm, which made it hard to hold objects (and the numbness made it even harder). My toes cramped at the least provocation, particularly when I was lying down in the evenings. I had infrequent but painful bouts of gastroesophageal reflux and gallbladder attacks and had to cut out all fried foods or suffer after I ate them. I became a bit unsteady on my feet and had to give up shoes with heels as I tended to wobble, but I thought maybe this was related to my back problems. My bladder got worse and worse, and sneezing or laughing proved a challenge.

The Onset of MS

My Early Symptoms
- Infertility
- Constipation
- Sinus infections
- Insomnia
- Numbness and pain in hands
- Loss of dexterity
- Fatigue
- Irritability
- Loss of vision
- Back pain
- Cramping of toes
- Gastroesophageal reflux and gallbladder attacks
- Loss of balance
- Incontinence

The Doctors I Saw
- Neurologist
- Orthopedist
- Ophthalmologist
- Urologist
- General practitioner
- Ob-gyn

I saw several doctors about these problems: an orthopedist for my back who did an X-ray and said I had irreversible arthritic degeneration about which nothing could be done; an eye doctor who said I had presbyopia (aging eyes) and gave me a prescription for reading glasses; a urologist for my incontinence who said age and childbirth had taken their toll and I should consider bladder surgery; and a general practitioner for my gallbladder and reflux problems who gave me prescriptions for various drugs to help with the symptoms.

I don't have to tell you how insidious this path is. I am willing to bet most of you reading this book have similar stories. We just keep going to one doctor after another with our lists of symptoms. We get one prescription after another and a referral to yet another specialist from our doctors, whose expressions say "hypochondriac," or worse…"crazy."

From Bad to Worse

It wasn't until I was 47 and the right side of my face began to get numb that I really got worried. I had Bell's palsy when I was 26 for about three months after a bad ear infection. I almost quit my job, as the paralysis made it difficult for me to talk. Fortunately, it resolved just as the neurologist said I was starting to have permanent nerve damage. Also, I choked on a small piece of meat at a dinner party and a friend had to do the Heimlich maneuver several times to clear it. A doctor friend sitting next to me (who by then had a knife in hand to do an emergency tracheotomy) said that I needed to get this looked at, as it was very unusual to choke on such a small object, and that it could be a sign of cancer or something else serious.

So between the fear of Bell's palsy returning and possible cancer, I went back to the neurologist to see what was going on. He spent five minutes with me and told me that I had MS. I still considered myself as basically healthy, so, needless to say, I was completely shocked. I guess I shouldn't have been, as my father had been diagnosed with Parkinson's disease 15 years earlier. After 10 years, his diagnosis had been changed to progressive supranuclear palsy (PSP). PSP is a fatal neurodegenerative brain disease that affects nerve cells that control walking, balance, mobility, vision, speech, and swallowing and is very similar to ALS (amyotrophic lateral sclerosis, or Lou Gehrig's disease) but clearly also has many of the same symptoms as MS. And, having seen my father experience slow and painful neurodegeneration, I was determined not to end up the same way.

> *Between the fear of Bell's palsy returning and possible cancer, I went back to the neurologist to see what was going on. He spent five minutes with me and told me that I had MS. I still considered myself as basically healthy, so, needless to say, I was completely shocked.*

The neurologist told me I needed an MRI and spinal tap in order to be sure that it was MS. He said they were both easy office procedures so I agreed to go ahead, hoping they would prove him wrong. Unfortunately, the spinal tap leaked afterward and for the next week I had to lie prone with crushing pain in my head and buzzing in my ears. My doctor had gone on vacation the day after I had the procedure done; my repeated calls to his office for help were answered by the nursing staff, who reassured me that this was common and told me that I would have to wait until he returned the next week to be seen. I found out later that the normal procedure when this happens is to apply a "blood patch," which essentially blocks the hole the spinal tap made and stops the spinal fluid from leaking. The situation finally resolved after a week, just as my doctor returned, but left a whole new raft of symptoms in its wake.

My fatigue was worse than ever and I had a very hard time concentrating and making sense out of simple things. I would have to reread pages in books over and over to try to make sense out of them; I would forget the story line and characters' names and have to flip back to the front of the book to figure out what was going on.

The trauma to my central nervous system (CNS) had been enough to cause significant deterioration in my eyesight. Now I could only see vague shapes out of my right eye. My fatigue was worse than ever and I had a very hard time concentrating and making sense out of simple things. I would have to reread pages in books over and over to try to make sense out of them; I would forget the story line and characters' names and have to flip back to the front of the book to figure out what was going on. Working with numbers was almost completely beyond me and my memory was terrible. I developed overwhelming back pain. It got so bad at night I had to prop four pillows under my legs so that they were essentially bent as if I were sitting in a chair. When I walked, I had to squat down and stretch my back out every 20 to 30 feet or it would completely seize up. All my other symptoms were greatly exacerbated and I found myself having to visit the emergency room on occasion to get catheterized because of the severity of my bladder problems or severe pain of one sort or another.

By this time, we had sold the company I had been running, and I was consulting only a day a week. I couldn't have continued in my job, anyway, with the fatigue and increasing cognitive confusion. Fortunately, this left me with time to focus solely on getting to the bottom of what was going on with my health.

Taking Control of My Health

I had worked in the biotech industry for years, running operations at a drug development company, so I knew how to conduct research projects and was conversant with scientific terminology. This background made it easier to figure out how to tackle such an intimidating project. As long as I started first thing in the morning, I could accomplish a lot before I got completely worn out and confused by early afternoon. At this point, I had no inkling that my endocrine system played a role in my health, but I was always convinced that I had to look at all the systems in my body to get to the bottom of what was going on. My neurologist had a myopic view of my health and seemed to believe my nervous system was not connected in any way to the rest of my body. This approach is effective if you need a specific surgery but is not a view destined to get to and fix the root cause of a problem.

> By this time, we had sold the company I had been running, and I was consulting only a day a week. I couldn't have continued in my job, anyway, with the fatigue and increasing cognitive confusion. Fortunately, this left me with time to focus solely on getting to the bottom of what was going on with my health.

Even though my earlier holistic efforts to reduce levels of toxic heavy metals and replace deficient vitamin and mineral levels hadn't had any effect on my symptoms, I still believed that identifying and correcting problems and deficiencies made the most sense in resolving them. I found a doctor who was open to this approach and embarked on a fact-finding mission.

I had everything tested that he and I could think of. We tested amino acid levels; did complex immune function tests; tested for every kind of virus and bacteria you can think of; looked at fatty acid levels, parasites, digestive function, allergies—you name it, we did it. And guess what? Everything looked awful.

I had no discernible immune function. We tested my levels of "complements," the natural defense mechanisms that protect our bodies from infections and perhaps tumors. Of the 23 tested, I had abnormal levels in 14. I had several viruses including Epstein-Barr. My lipid peroxidation level was elevated (this is when lipid damage results in production of free radicals). I had flourishing bacteria and gut dysfunction, which resulted in my not being able to absorb nutrients from the food I was eating. I was completely under the low end of the test range in 19 of the 20 amino acids. This came as no surprise, as I was obviously not digesting much and amino acids are derived from the protein we eat. I had stopped eating meat because I couldn't digest it. I ate a small amount of chicken but mainly existed on simple carbs like pasta, as well as some vegetables. Subsequently, I have found research that shows that meat negatively affects the body when the thyroid isn't functioning. Studies show that when the thyroids of meat-eating animals are removed and they are fed meat, they die. If they are fed other types of food, they are fine.[1] This probably explains why so many of us with MS find ourselves eating less and less meat as our conditions progress.

> *At this point, I had no inkling that my endocrine system played a role in my health, but I was always convinced that I had to look at all the systems in my body to get to the bottom of what was going on.*

As depressing as I found all these lab test results, at least they gave me somewhere to start. I immediately scheduled a series of amino acid IV infusions to try to get my levels up. Amino acids are the building blocks of protein in our bodies and are essential to synthesize proteins, enzymes, and some hormones and neurotransmitters. Certain amino acids (e.g., arginine, histidine, ornithine, lysine, methionine, and phenylalanine) are thought to stimulate the release of growth hormone, insulin, and cortisol and thereby promote the anabolic processes that build up organs and tissues. I had a great response to the IV and felt wonderful for two days afterward. My fatigue disappeared, I slept well, and my mind was clear all day for the first time in a long time. I had an amino acid drip once a month for about six months, but unfortunately, in every case the effect was temporary.

I tried several other alternative therapies as well as one of the FDA-approved drugs, Copaxone, which gave me large, swollen, painful lumps at the injection site and didn't affect my symptoms at all. I gave it up after three months.

The Greatest Discovery: Hormones

The next thing I did after the lab testing, and while trying these new therapies, was sit down and look at all my symptoms in a logical, systematic way. When I

> *I had a great response to the IV and felt wonderful for two days afterward. My fatigue disappeared, I slept well, and my mind was clear all day for the first time in a long time.*
>
> *I had an amino acid drip once a month for about six months, but unfortunately, in every case the effect was temporary.*

The next thing I did after the lab testing, and while trying these new therapies, was sit down and look at all my symptoms in a logical, systematic way. When I finished, everything pointed me in the direction of my endocrine system.

finished, everything pointed me in the direction of my endocrine system.

The traditional symptoms of MS include chronic fatigue, sleep problems, muscle stiffness and cramping, neuralgia, bladder and bowel problems, sexual dysfunction, coordination and balance issues, difficulty walking, numbness, vision changes, gastroesophageal reflux, and cognitive impairment. I suffered from all of these symptoms. When I researched them on the computer, I found out that amino acids stimulate production of hormones and also that all of my symptoms were those of hormone deficiency. I thought maybe the reason that I had so much symptom relief from the amino acid therapy was due to a transient increase in hormone production. I also saw striking similarities between MS and symptoms of perimenopause. Both conditions have similar symptoms at around the same age. I called my doctor, filled him in on what I had found, and went to get my hormone levels tested.

I had my levels of estrogen, progesterone, and thyroid hormones tested. My estrogen and progesterone levels were very low, so I began taking prescription bio-identical estrogen and progesterone. These are biologically identical to the hormones we make in our bodies—atom for atom. It made much more sense to me to put substances in my body that it had made all my life (particularly when I was young and healthy) and knew just what to do with. My thyroid levels were all in the "normal" range, which I thought was odd as so many of my symptoms seemed to point to low thyroid. The estrogen and progesterone replacement reduced the severity of my symptoms, especially bladder problems and fatigue, so I knew I was finally on to something; however, many of my symptoms remained.

> The estrogen and progesterone replacement reduced the severity of my symptoms, especially bladder problems and fatigue, so I knew I was finally on to something; however, many of my symptoms remained.

I continued research on the rest of the endocrine system and also read up on thyroid testing. I soon realized that thyroid testing is completely confusing and there are a lot of variables to evaluate to get an accurate picture of your thyroid health. I added a couple of other thyroid tests and went to get retested. Sure enough, when I finally had the whole picture, it was obvious I was completely deficient in one of the thyroid hormones that is virtually never tested: something called T3 (more about this in Chapter 5)— unfortunately the type of thyroid hormone most biologically active in our bodies. When I learned this I talked to my doctor, who remained uncomfortable about prescribing thyroid hormones to me, as the "normal tests" were in "normal ranges." But in a conversation with my mother around this time, I learned that she had started on thyroid medicine at 46 (as had

> *After a week of serious anxiety, feeling myself slipping back into MS, I returned to my research. Why would I have gotten rid of all my symptoms only to have them return again within a month?*

her mother and sister). This family history finally convinced him to give me a trial course of thyroid therapy.

The thyroid hormones made the most profound difference in my symptoms of "MS." They resolved the fatigue that had plagued me for more than five years, I slept beautifully every night, my back pain went away completely, my vision started to come back, my mind was clear and my memory restored, energy, bladder, libido, digestion—all completely resolved. It was a miracle…or was it?

Three weeks after I reached my optimal dose of thyroid medication, my miraculous "cure" disappeared and I started to get my symptoms back. It began with fatigue and brain fog. I definitely didn't feel the same. Then one thing after another reappeared. I started to panic. I had been sure I was finally better. After a week of serious anxiety, feeling myself slipping back into MS, I returned to my research. Why would I have gotten rid of all my symptoms only to have them return again within a month? Fortunately, I came upon the answer within a couple of days. It was my adrenal function.

Your adrenals are closely linked to your thyroid. Think of it like this: When low thyroid function affects your body's metabolism, it moves in slow motion and all your organs and glands function in slow motion, as well. When your thyroid speeds up, everything else is suddenly asked to speed up, too. Because the rest of your endocrine system has been affected by low thyroid function for a long time, it's incapable of much additional effort and has a hard time keeping up with the higher demand. This is what happened to my adrenals, something called adrenal fatigue (see Chapter 6 for more information).

When I had my adrenal function tested (which is done by a lab test measuring cortisol several times a day), it was clear that my adrenals were seriously compromised and the only solution for me was to replace my cortisol levels with low doses of bio-identical cortisol four times a day. The first day I used the cortisol, I felt I'd rediscovered my health—and so ends this long saga.

As of this writing, I have felt great for more than two years. Am I cured? Unfortunately, no. When I stop my hormones even for a day, my symptoms come back. Maybe they're not as bad, but severe nonetheless. But at 54, I am healthier than most of my friends who've never had serious medical conditions. All my lab tests look great, so all systems are humming along—and best of all, I feel completely well again. I believe some of the aging processes have been reversed, too, as I no longer need glasses to read—no more presbyopia!

The thyroid hormones made the most profound difference in my symptoms of "MS." They resolved the fatigue that had plagued me for more than five years, I slept beautifully every night, my back pain went away completely, my vision started to come back, my mind was clear and my memory restored, energy, bladder, libido, digestion—all completely resolved. It was a miracle...or was it?

And the Rest Is History

The interesting thing is that after I figured out what was happening and resolved my symptoms by replacing the deficient hormones, I started to find confirmation of this connection everywhere. It's

It was clear that my adrenals were seriously compromised and the only solution for me was to replace my cortisol levels with low doses of bio-identical cortisol four times a day. The first day I used the cortisol, I felt I'd rediscovered my health.

become more and more surprising to me that no one else seems to have figured it out. I have taken to reading and researching scientific literature from the late 1800s and early 1900s; the medical world was a very different place before it became completely dependent on pharmaceutical drugs to treat the symptoms of illness. In a more recent book, *The Thyroid and Its Diseases,* I found a particularly interesting list of symptoms of hypothyroidism including headache, numbness, carpal tunnel syndrome, lack of coordination, deafness, tinnitus, vertigo, sleep apnea, depression, psychoses, and bi-polar disorder.

It also states that two signs of hypothyroidism are prolonged evoked potentials (a test that measures the time it takes for nerves to respond to stimulation) and elevated cerebral spinal fluid protein and immunoglobulin G (IgG) levels. The "definitive" diagnosis for MS is made primarily on the results of these two tests, as well as detection of lesions in the brain and spinal cord by an MRI.[2]

It's also well-known that hypothyroidism can cause lesions in the brain. With all the test results for MS and low thyroid function being the same, could it be that some cases of MS are really just hypothyroidism? In my case, and in many others I've seen, it is. It's important to realize, though, that by the time we get the severe symptoms of "MS," we've usually experienced damage to other endocrine glands, as well, so it's important to evaluate all your hormone levels at the same time. With sophisticated hormone blood testing now available at most labs, testing levels of these important hormones should be the first thing that's done when symptoms of neurological dysfunction are detected.

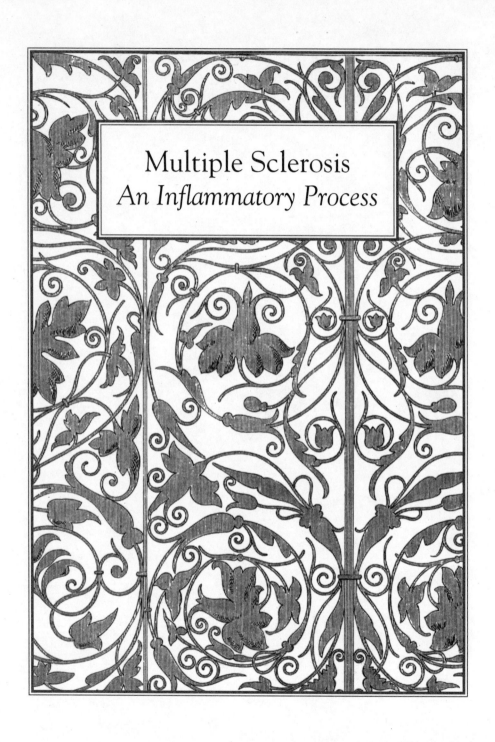

Multiple Sclerosis
An Inflammatory Process

II

What Is Multiple Sclerosis?

Multiple sclerosis is a confusing disease. It's thought that our variable and distressing symptoms are caused by the loss of myelin, the fatty substance that coats our nerves. This process occurs in the central nervous system and prevents our nerves from conducting impulses as they should. Pockets of scar tissue, which are called plaques or lesions, form in these areas of nerve damage in the brain and spinal cord, thus the name multiple sclerosis meaning "many scars."

After this, everything gets murky. To begin with, a lot of other conditions can cause these plaques. And the confusion surrounding MS continues, as there's no unanimous agreement as to what causes it. Many speculate that the loss of nerve myelination, called demyelination, is caused by an autoimmune process in which the body's immune system attacks its own healthy tissue by mistake while trying to get rid of some foreign object such as a bacteria or virus. This theory has spurred drug companies to develop the current class of immune-modulating drugs to treat MS. These medications (Avonex, Betaseron, and Rebif) resemble the natural substance called interferon, which your immune system produces in response to disease. It's not completely clear how these medications work, but it's known that they affect the immune system to help fight viral infections and prevent inflammation.

It may well be that there is some autoimmune element in MS, but because there's no known way to cure an autoimmune disease, let's look at the process that we know causes the demyelination that wreaks so much havoc on our bodies—inflammation. Everyone seems to agree on one thing: MS is widely acknowledged to be an inflammatory disease of the central nervous system. When I set out to solve the riddle of my MS, my thinking was that if this inflammatory process could be resolved, then the demyelination would also be resolved and my symptoms would go with it.

Everyone seems to agree on one thing: MS is widely acknowledged to be an inflammatory disease of the central nervous system. When I set out to solve the riddle of my MS, my thinking was that if this inflammatory process could be resolved, then the demyelination would also be resolved and my symptoms would go with it.

Inflammation's involvement in demyelination has been studied extensively and understood well for many years. But for some peculiar reason, this concept has not been followed to its logical conclusion: finding out what basic biological events cause inflammation and resolving them.

Extensive research has shown that loss of key hormones starts the inflammatory cascade of events that can end in neurodegenerative disease. We need to consider that if loss of hormones causes the problem, then maybe replacing these natural substances to treat our symptoms makes a lot of sense. When our levels of estrogen, testosterone, progesterone, thyroid, cortisol, and growth hormone are robust, we have little inflammatory activity in our bodies—no obvious signs such as aches, pains, swollen joints, or allergies. And, not surprisingly, when we add them back, the aches and pains and other symptoms of inflammation disappear. Why use foreign substances that may have unpleasant side effects to treat individual symptoms when there are naturally occurring substances available that your body knows exactly what to do with? I never advocate that anyone stop a drug that a doctor has prescribed; I merely suggest that we apply common sense in trying to get to the root of and fix our problems.

Inflammation...How Did We Get Here?

Our world is getting more and more inflammatory. Just watch the ads on TV and you'll realize that many Americans have significant inflammation, as evidenced by all the advertisements for various anti-inflammatory drugs: statin drugs for our arteries, nonsteroidal anti-inflammatory drugs (NSAIDs) and COX-2 inhibitors for our joints, not to mention Claritin and the like for all those allergies. These drugs may help with short-term, isolated instances of inflammation, but the bottom line is that hormones reduce inflammation throughout our bodies.

> *We need to consider that if loss of hormones causes the problem, then maybe replacing these natural substances to treat our symptoms makes a lot of sense.*

Think of your youth: Did your joints swell up or ache after a vigorous game of volleyball or basketball? Could you jog without having to pay the price later? Did hugging your cat used to result in itching and sneezing? Could you shop at a cosmetic counter in a department store without having to flee after five minutes, eyes streaming? Inflammation causes these insidious changes, and you might be surprised to learn that many symptoms can be resolved by adjusting your hormone levels to fit the profile of the young and healthy person that you used to be.

But before we jump to the solution, let's look at how we got here to begin with. Inflammation is a necessary thing in its place. It's how your body responds to illness or injury. When you are in a critical condition, your body releases inflammatory substances to defend yourself, which keeps you alive. This is fine for short-term emergencies. But what happens when the inflammation is chronic? Easy: degeneration and death.

Inflammation causes these insidious changes, and you might be surprised to learn that many symptoms can be resolved by adjusting your hormone levels to fit the profile of the young and healthy person that you used to be.

If we look at our bodies in the context of how we lived centuries ago, we see that many of the biochemical actions that are killing us now were necessary to survival back then. We didn't always have antibiotics and the like, so when we had an acute infection, inflammation was what got us through. It mobilized our defenses and fought off bacterial and viral invaders. Life is very different today, and our inflammation is often caused by completely different things, like diet, lifestyle, and chronic stress. The biochemical mechanisms that respond to these things now shorten our lives.

If we look at our bodies in the context of how we lived centuries ago, we see that many of the biochemical actions that are killing us now were necessary to survival back then.

The Hormone Connection

MS research has been focusing on ways to stop and treat the symptoms of damage done by inflammation. But what's been overlooked is that all of our "sex hormones"—in other words, those that are made in ovaries in women and testicles in men—as well as hormones made in other glands, like the thyroid and adrenals, do a remarkable job of reducing inflammation, along with the demyelination and excess immune activity that inflammation causes.

It's important to say that I do not believe that MS is caused solely by deficient hormones. If this were the case, all women would have MS after menopause. There are clearly many factors involved. Genetics and the environment both play a role. Environmental factors include the chemicals, bacteria, and viruses you're exposed to; the food you eat; the substances you use; exercise, sleep, and stress; and every other aspect of your daily life. All these factors affect your hormone levels and can also permanently compromise your endocrine glands. At the present time, we have only one way to ensure optimal health for the remainder of our lives: Evaluate endocrine function and replace any hormones that are low or out of balance.

At the present time, we have only one way to ensure optimal health for the remainder of our lives: Evaluate endocrine function and replace any hormones that are low or out of balance.

> Your endocrine system is made up of nine glands that regulate and control an extraordinary number of your body's functions and make more than 100 hormones. These glands are the hypothalamus, pituitary, thyroid, parathyroid, adrenal, thymus, pancreas, pineal, and reproductive—ovaries and testes.

We have only to apply common sense to see the connection between hormone levels and MS. There's an obvious relationship between age, hormones, and the progression of MS:

- MS is approximately four times more prevalent in women than in men. Ovaries shut down at menopause and testicles don't, so women lose much more of their hormone levels (and much earlier) than men do.
- The mean age of onset of MS is 32. Hormone production in the ovaries drops significantly in the mid-30s, closely paralleling the typical time MS starts.
- The increased levels of sex hormones produced during pregnancy are associated with a significant reduction in symptoms of MS, while symptoms often worsen postpartum, when there's a significant drop in hormone levels.
- The first clinical symptoms of MS develop after puberty, when hormone issues begin.
- The disease moves to the "secondary progressive" phase, characterized by chronic, progressively worsening symptoms, in the same general time frame as hormone levels decline. Of MS cases, 50% become progressive within 10 to 15 years, and an additional 40% do so within 25 years of onset. MS generally progresses faster in those who experience their first symptoms after age 40.[1]
- The symptoms of MS are also well-known symptoms of hormone deficiency. Look at the list and then at the inhabitants of your local retirement home: numbness and tingling, chronic fatigue, bladder and bowel problems, balance problems and decreased coordination; vision abnormalities, cognitive impairment, sleep

> *There's an obvious relationship between age, hormones, and the progression of MS.*

Lauren's Story

Lauren is a 45-year-old woman who was diagnosed with multiple sclerosis at age 39. Her first symptoms were of numbness and loss of feeling in her right leg and visual disturbances that began in her early 30s but were intermittent until age 39. At this time they became chronic and she was diagnosed with MS. Other symptoms were optic neuritis, chronic fatigue, anxiety, depression, cognitive dysfunction, neuralgia, sleep disturbances, bladder difficulties, tinnitus, sexual dysfunction, bowel problems, chronic infections, allergies, and breathing problems.

Lauren's estrogen and progesterone levels were very low and she was started on estrogen and progesterone replacement in February 2007. Her thyroid tests were all low but within "normal" ranges. Her doctor decided to wait and see if the estrogen and progesterone resolved her symptoms before doing anything about her thyroid. Although her symptoms got better in the next two months, she still had breathing, cognitive, and hearing problems, among others, so her doctor decided to try thyroid therapy. The results were exciting—all her other symptoms started to resolve. The only symptom that didn't totally resolve was her fatigue. Her doctor measured her cortisol levels and found them to be very low. She was started on very low dose cortisol four times a day and almost immediately her fatigue was gone. She had been unable to function in the afternoons for almost 10 years and she finds she can now function through the evenings.

problems, gastroesophageal reflux, emotional problems, mood swings, depression, sexual dysfunction, muscle stiffness and cramping, and neuralgia. Do you see the similarities? Neither of us has any hormones left.

All this evidence, albeit anecdotal, shows a clear connection between hormones and MS. Fortunately we do not have to go on supposition and detective work alone. There have been hundreds, if not thousands, of well-documented studies that support this hypothesis. In subsequent chapters we'll look at these studies and the role that individual hormones play in neurological health.

> All this evidence, albeit anecdotal, shows a clear connection between hormones and MS. Fortunately we do not have to go on supposition and detective work alone. There have been hundreds, if not thousands, of well-documented studies that support this hypothesis.

Connections in Your Brain

The brain is just as affected by the harmful consequences of inflammation as the rest of our bodies. Actually, the brain is less able to protect itself from inflammation than are other parts of the body. This is why we see devastating effects created by diseases like Alzheimer's, in which the brain is "on fire." When our brains are working as they should, they're constantly being replenished and rebuilt—a process called remyelination.

A brief explanation: Brains are made up of cells called neurons and glia. The glia, named by a German scientist for the word "glue," come in small and large sizes: microglia and macroglia, respectively. Microglia cells drive your body's response to inflammation when you have an injury or infection. Think of Pac-Man. (Are any of you that old?) To help, these Pac-Men travel to the site of an injury to eat up damaged tissue by using chemicals called cytokines. Unfortunately, this is a double-edged sword because microglia can generate substances that cause further injury by making the site of the original injury larger and worsening the inflammation and neurological dysfunction.

The macroglia cells, on the other hand, maintain and replenish the myelin sheaths that surround your nerves. Macroglia come in four different cell types: Schwann cells, oligodendrocytes, astrocytes, and ependymal cells. In the interest of getting through this, let's stick to oligodendrocytes and Schwann cells, which are critical in MS because they're responsible for keeping nerve axons healthy and coated with myelin. Axons are the connectors between neurons that transmit nerve impulses. When axons lose

Pathways of Immunity—T1 and T2

In talking to your doctor or during the course of your research, you might have encountered the terms "T1" and "T2" in relation to MS. T cells are lymphocytes, a type of white blood cell made in your thymus gland that is very important to optimal functioning of your immune system. Simply put, T1 cells are pro-inflammatory and T2 are anti-inflammatory. MS is basically a T1 pro-inflammatory condition, as are all autoimmune diseases. Interestingly enough, aging and hormone deficiency also cause us to travel down this T1 path. Studies have shown that replacing deficient hormones can shift you back to T2 dominance and increase anti-inflammatory activity. Testosterone is key in causing this shift, but other important hormones involved are progesterone, estrogen, and vitamin D (which is actually a hormone, not a vitamin—more in Chapter 7).

Microglia and macroglia cells have hormone receptors, which respond to progesterone, estrogen, testosterone, growth hormone, thyroid, and cortisol. Without the right amount and balance of these hormones, demyelination ensues, picks up speed, and we start to see nerve communication break down and the symptoms of MS begin.

their myelin coating, the impulses can't make the leap from one nerve to the next—and that's when we start losing our ability to walk and experience all those other symptoms we're so familiar with.[2]

The key thing to remember out of this section (as I'm determined to make all this information useful to you) is that both microglia and macroglia cells have hormone receptors, which respond to progesterone, estrogen, testosterone, growth hormone, thyroid, and cortisol. Without the right amount and balance of these hormones, demyelination ensues and picks up speed, and we start to see nerve communication break down and the symptoms of MS begin.[3]

Parkinson's Disease and Inflammation

Dopamine is a neurotransmitter critical for coordinating movement, and the loss of dopamine neurons triggers symptoms of Parkinson's disease. Progesterone, testosterone, and estrogen have been found to protect dopaminergic neurons against degeneration.[4] Loss of adequate levels of these hormones may play a role in the development of the disease. Also, studies have shown the risk of its occurrence is increased in women who have an early menopause, which causes a steep drop in levels of estrogen, progesterone, and testosterone.[5] People with Parkinson's have been shown to have significantly elevated inflammatory markers, suggesting that it may be an inflammatory disease like MS. An even more exciting study, with 140,000 participants, showed that people who had been taking anti-inflammatory NSAIDs for 14 to 18 years had a 45% reduction in risk of Parkinson's disease.[6]

Effects on Your Body

In multiple sclerosis, the myelin sheath around the nerve axon becomes damaged and dramatically slows the speed of nerve transmissions. Signals throughout your body are affected. You must have good communication between your brain, the rest of your central nervous system, and your peripheral nerves for your sensory and motor functions to work. Longer axons are necessary for motor and sensory neurons to be able to carry information, so they're more dependent on the insulating myelin for transmission. Therefore, the destruction of the myelin most affects them.

Many of the common symptoms of MS are examples of the failure of sensory or motor neurons to effectively send signals from your brain and spinal cord to your muscles and nerves. These include problems with vision, coordination, gait, motor reflexes, strength, sensation, speech, swallowing, bladder control, and sexual function. The numbness and tingling we get happens when sensory neurons that carry information from your sense organs to the brain are damaged. Our vision problems can occur when the motor neurons that control eye movement and visual coordination are affected or when the sensory optic nerve is damaged or inflamed. Sexual dysfunction is the bane of almost everyone with MS. It can stem from damage to the motor neurons that control physical arousal or to the sensory axons that transmit information about sexual sensation.

> *Many of the common symptoms of MS are examples of the failure of sensory or motor neurons to effectively send signals from your brain and spinal cord to your muscles and nerves.*

Some symptoms are believed to be caused by the physical lesions in the brain. The cerebellum is responsible for maintaining your sense of

MS affects your brain's ability to process data, so cognitive difficulties are common.

equilibrium, so lesions in this area can affect your balance and spatial perception. MS affects your brain's ability to process data, so cognitive difficulties are common. These include problems with information processing or abstract reasoning, memory loss, decreased language ability (which results in our never being able to find the words we want), and lessened intellectual function.

What Can You Do to Combat Inflammation?

Because we know that MS is an inflammatory condition, we need to make reducing inflammation our top priority. The fact is that there's a lot we can do to control it. When we get a diagnosis of multiple sclerosis, we feel completely powerless to do anything because we're told it's incurable and progressive. Picking out a wheelchair and thinking about long-term care options aren't anybody's idea of taking charge of the situation and making things happen. The exciting time comes when you realize that MS is just a constellation of symptoms indicating that something is going wrong and needs to be fixed—not a death sentence. You can start today to make the changes that will hopefully restore your health.

The exciting time comes when you realize that MS is just a constellation of symptoms indicating that something is going wrong and needs to be fixed—not a death sentence. You can start today to make the changes that will hopefully restore your health.

Test and Balance Your Endocrine System

The number one solution to stopping the downward spiral that inflammation causes in the body is rebuilding the endocrine system by measuring and replacing deficient hormones. I won't go into specifics now, as later chapters are dedicated to specific hormones, but there are other important things you can do to reduce inflammation.

Look at Your Insulin Levels and Lose Excess Weight

The first step is to get rid of your abdominal fat. This fat essentially becomes a dangerous organ that makes its own inflammatory substances and affects nerve health. I know this seems easier said than done—but not necessarily. Abdominal fat comes from several things, among them high levels of blood sugar (glucose), insulin, and cortisol and low levels of sex hormones and growth hormone.

When our insulin levels stay too high for too long (generally because we eat too many simple carbs, such as bread, sugar, and the like), it results in something called insulin resistance. This is a condition in which the body stops responding to insulin correctly and ends up putting weight around our middle. Insulin resistance goes hand in hand with elevated cortisol levels. Cortisol is our "stress hormone," which means it's a hormone that the body makes when it perceives some threat or stressor. Strangely enough, it doesn't matter if this is a physical threat such as infection, injury, or an attack, or if it's just a perceived threat to our happiness or safety. It could be as simple as a demanding boss or an argumentative teenager. These emotional "threats" also trigger your body into making more cortisol than it really needs.

The number one solution to stopping the downward spiral that inflammation causes in the body is rebuilding the endocrine system by measuring and replacing deficient hormones.

Chronic excess cortisol results in compromised immune function and then—you guessed it—more inflammation. Elevated cortisol also prevents estrogen and testosterone from doing their jobs, one of which is

Causes of Inflammation

Be alert for some of these other factors that cause inflammation. Many of them are diet related:

- Deficient levels of any hormone. Get levels measured and supplement deficiencies.
- Free radical exposure from the environment (things like X-rays and pollution). Try to avoid exposure whenever possible and see Chapter 8 for suggested vitamins and minerals to minimize damage.
- Large amounts of animal fats rich in arachidonic acid produce omega-6 fatty acids, which can be inflammatory. Consumption of omega-6 oils should be controlled, whether they're derived from animals or made from soy, cottonseed, or safflower. Try to eat red meat no more than four to five times a week, and if possible, buy meat from free-range cows that have not been fed antibiotics or hormones.
- Excess adipose fat (generally around your middle) becomes an inflammation-producing organ in and of itself. Get rid of it.
- Too much food. Overeating produces inflammatory substances.[7]
- Something called advanced glycation endproducts (AGEs). AGEs can be formed outside of your body by heating or cooking sugars with fats or proteins at high heats; or, inside the body, through normal metabolism and aging. These AGEs create oxidative and peroxidative stress and are toxic to your body. Try to boil, steam, or poach foods instead of broiling, frying, or grilling, and keep your stove set to as low a temperature as possible.

to maintain the hourglass female shape and the muscled, trim male shape. After years of too much cortisol, we all end up looking like we have 20-pound fryers strapped to our waists.

Getting levels of glucose, insulin, and cortisol tested gives you a lot of good information. If they are elevated, you have somewhere to start. Dropping levels of estrogen in women and testosterone in both men and women are common causes of high cortisol, so it may be as easy as supplementing these hormones. See Chapters 6 and 7 for more ideas on reducing cortisol, glucose, and insulin.

Find and Treat Infections

Infections caused by viruses and bacteria can also be a source of chronic systemic inflammation, so eliminating infections is important. Even a subclinical tooth infection can be a constant source of inflammatory activity and take a big toll on our bodies and nerves.[8]

Key Points

- MS is caused by inflammation that results in demyelination of the nerves.
- The symptoms of MS and the symptoms of hormone deficiency are the same.
- There is an obvious relationship between age, hormones, and the progression of MS.
- Endocrine glands such as ovaries, testes, thyroid, and adrenals make hormones that control inflammation. When you lose these key hormones, inflammation results. Replacing these hormones in a way that mimics your youthful hormone profile may result in amelioration of both inflammation and the symptoms of MS.

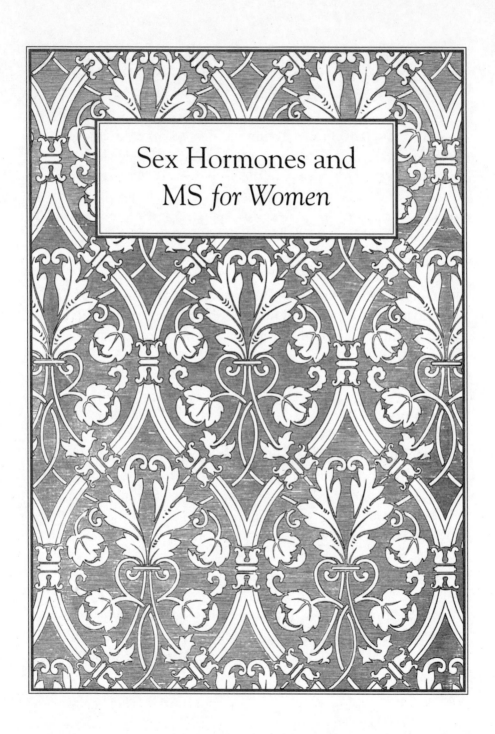

Sex Hormones and MS *for Women*

III

Why Are My Ovaries Important?

The similarities between the progression of MS and women's progressive loss of hormones are obvious, with this coincidence most conspicuous in our ovarian function. Men's levels of testosterone generally decline gradually as they age, but women lose 90% of their estrogen and progesterone production within a short two-year period at menopause. Menopause is also when many women with MS are hit the hardest, and the "progressive" stage of the disease begins with symptoms becoming chronic.[1]

Our ovaries produce "sex hormones," including estrogen, progesterone, and testosterone. Tied to our menstrual cycle, estrogen and progesterone are produced in a cyclic fashion. In the first two weeks of the cycle, an egg ripens until approximately day 13, when ovulation occurs and it's released for fertilization. Estrogen levels increase throughout this time and reach their peak when we ovulate. Progesterone is only produced in high levels after ovulation, as it's made by the empty egg sac left behind after the egg is released. Estrogen causes cell proliferation, and progesterone tempers it. So, if you don't ovulate, this balance is thrown off, causing problems as minor as sore breasts and as major as increased risk of neurological problems and cancer.

> *Is it just a coincidence that the mean age for diagnosis of MS is 32—just as many women experience their first significant drop in hormone levels?*

You're born with your lifetime supply of eggs, so although you start out with about 2 million, by your mid- to late 30s you only have about 3% left. Every month when you ovulate, you reduce a bit more of this supply. This decrease starts to lower the levels of all of your ovarian hormones as early as your 30s. Is it just a coincidence that the mean age for diagnosis of MS is 32—just as many women experience their first significant drop in hormone levels?

Many women have inherited genetically lower levels of ovarian hormones to start with and tend to lose estrogen, progesterone, and testosterone earlier than women with naturally higher levels, which may explain why some women get MS symptoms earlier than others. All women have genetically programmed levels of hormones, and breast size offers a good clue to individual levels. High estrogen levels cause more stimulation to breast tissue, which is rich in estrogen receptors, and the result is larger breasts. Clinical studies have shown that women with large breasts and narrow waists have much higher levels of progesterone and estrogen than do other women. The voluptuous women in the study had 26% higher overall estrogen levels, and were 37% higher at ovulation.[2]

Progesterone and estrogen ebb and flow during the normal menstrual cycle. The following chart illustrates their pattern.

Estrogen and Progesterone in the Menstrual Cycle

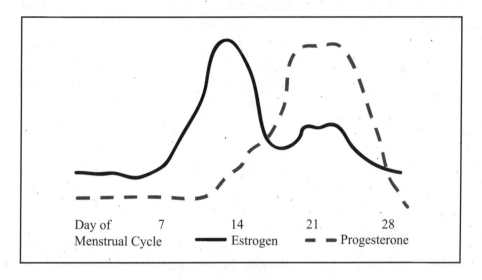

This chart makes it easy to visualize the problem that cycles without ovulation can cause. The production of progesterone requires ovulation, so when you don't ovulate, the healthy, buoyant peaks of estrogen at ovulation and of progesterone in the second half of your cycle don't occur. This lack of ovulation can affect nerve health profoundly, as both estrogen and progesterone are critical in nerve health and remyelination. Most women can attest to the importance of progesterone, as they experience sleeping and mood problems, headaches, brain fog, cognitive difficulty, and sore breasts when they don't ovulate.

All of our sex hormones are important in myelination and overall nerve health. Many

> *All of our sex hormones are important in myelination and overall nerve health. Many studies have shown that they can affect the course of multiple sclerosis, but for some reason mainstream researchers don't seem to have connected the dots yet.*

studies have shown that they can affect the course of multiple sclerosis, but for some reason mainstream researchers don't seem to have connected the dots yet. Sex hormones in both men and women have a huge effect on MS. The same hormones have different consequences for men and women, although the basic functions of the individual hormones are much the same for everyone.[3]

Estrogen is currently being used in clinical studies to treat multiple sclerosis, so it's baffling that very few in the medical world seem to know that supplementing estrogen results not only in resolving symptoms of MS in women, but that it actually gets rid of inflammatory lesions in the central nervous system.

The Power of Estrogen

Estrogen is currently being used in clinical studies to treat multiple sclerosis, so it's baffling that very few in the medical world seem to know that supplementing estrogen results not only in resolving symptoms of MS in women, but that it actually *gets rid of* inflammatory lesions in the central nervous system.[4] Research has proven that treatment with estrogen can have a significant positive effect on MS in women, as well as on other autoimmune diseases such as rheumatoid arthritis.[5] Most scientists and doctors agree that pregnancy resolves MS symptoms, so it should be no surprise that treatment with estrogen at levels less than or equal to those in pregnancy have been found to significantly alter the course of the disease.[6] I started having symptoms of low estrogen at 43. Estrogen and progesterone were the first hormones I supplemented when I began to correct my hormone deficiencies, and they made a huge difference in my symptoms.

When estrogen levels drop, most women feel it. Some may make it through perimenopause and menopause feeling great, but they're a small minority. Most of us experience such things as hot flashes and night sweats; sleeping problems; vaginal dryness and loss of elasticity of vaginal tissue; more frequent urinary tract infections and urinary incontinence; changes in mood, or depression; loss of sexual desire and function; memory problems; skin changes including loss of collagen and moisture, thinner skin, and wrinkles; loss of breast tissue and firmness; increased cholesterol levels; and bone loss. Estrogen is also necessary for the body to make use of progesterone. It creates the progesterone receptors necessary for your body to effectively utilize it.

> *Estrogen and progesterone were the first hormones I supplemented when I began to correct my hormone deficiencies, and they made a huge difference in my symptoms.*

Progesterone: The Overlooked Hormone

Since its discovery centuries ago, progesterone has been thought of primarily as a pregnancy hormone—it was even named for "pro-gestation." The empty egg sac produces this hormone after it releases an egg at ovulation, so it's abundant only in the last two weeks of the menstrual cycle. Many women stop ovulating regularly in their mid- to late 30s. This not only causes an imbalance between progesterone and estrogen, it also prevents the body from performing the numerous important activities for which progesterone is responsible. Researchers have now found progesterone receptors all over the body, indicating progesterone's widespread effects. Areas with progesterone receptors include the reproductive organs, urinary tract, bones, breasts, skin, hair, heart, blood vessels, mucous membranes, and brain.[7] In the world of neurodegenerative disease, its most important function is remyelinating your nerves each and every month.

Critical Functions of Estrogen

Almost every function in your body depends on estrogen, as it causes cells and neurons to grow. Here are some of its many additional benefits:

Nerve Health
- Increases oxygenation and blood flow to the brain
- Causes nerve growth and maintains nerve function for increased cognitive and memory function
- Enhances magnesium uptake and utilization for optimal nerve health
- Necessary for the deep, restorative phase of sleep that repairs nerves

Brain
- Stimulates the production of an enzyme that prevents Alzheimer's disease
- Aids in the formation of neurotransmitters in the brain—serotonin, for example, which decreases depression, irritability, anxiety, and pain sensitivity
- Helps maintain memory

Muscle and Bone
- Helps to maintain muscle
- Maintains bone density, slows loss of bone to help prevent osteoporosis

Vision
- Prevents macular degeneration
- Keeps eye tissues moist
- Helps maintain good eyesight [8]

Mood
- Responsible for cheerful mood—prevents depression

Heart
- Keeps heart healthy and helps protect against coronary artery disease. Helps to maintain the elasticity of arteries. Decreases accumulation of plaque on the arteries.
- Decreases blood pressure
- Decreases LDL cholesterol

Reproduction
- Controls the menstrual cycle and prepares for conception

Skin
- Maintains collagen and moisture to keep skin firm, elastic, smooth, thick, and unwrinkled. Without hormone replacement, approximately 30% of skin collagen is lost in the first five years after menopause.

Bladder
- Maintains bladder, vagina, and genitals for optimal sex drive and bladder function

Overall Health
- Reduces inflammation
- Supports immune function
- Keeps tissues moist
- Important for thyroid function
- Necessary to create progesterone receptors
- Creates the female shape in breasts, hips, and pelvis
- Prevents excess hair growth in women
- Relieves hot flashes and night sweats
- Improves insulin sensitivity
- Increases energy
- Decreases the risk of colon cancer

Why Is Progesterone Important?

- Important in memory and cognitive function
- Stimulates bone growth and helps prevent osteoporosis
- Protects your heart by maintaining vascular tone and optimal cholesterol levels
- Helps prevent blood clots to prevent strokes
- Ensures optimal immune function
- Regulates fluid balance
- Necessary for sex drive and function
- Normalizes sleep
- Balances estrogen-induced cellular proliferation and helps prevent endometrial and breast cancer
- Necessary for emotional equilibrium and prevents mood swings
- Critical to effective adrenal and thyroid function
- Sensitizes estrogen receptors
- Maintains blood sugar control
- Is a precursor, or building block, for other hormones
- Necessary for reproductive function and normal menstrual cycles
- Adequate progesterone results in less water retention in the brain. For this reason, some neurosurgeons use progesterone injections before surgery to prevent swelling due to water retention.

Progesterone's Role in MS

It's surprising that progesterone is ignored in the treatment of MS because a large amount of research is available showing its vital role in myelination and remyelination. Progesterone holds enormous potential for effectively treating MS, as it both preserves and restores the integrity of myelin sheaths, which enable fast and efficient conduction of electrical impulses along nerve fibers. It has been shown to actually regenerate nerves after lesions have occurred.[9] It's thought to protect and regenerate nerves by accelerating the formation of new myelin sheaths, and by increasing survival of existing neurons.[10]

> *Progesterone holds enormous potential for effectively treating MS, as it both preserves and restores the integrity of myelin sheaths, which enable fast and efficient conduction of electrical impulses along nerve fibers. It has been shown to actually regenerate nerves after lesions have occurred.*

We lose myelin as we age, and the myelin sheath that remains becomes more and more compromised. Myelin sheaths in the brain actually start to break down and become irregular. We lose white matter and our ability to remyelinate nerves decreases.[11] Myelin disruption occurs in men and women even during normal aging, and a large number of studies have shown that progesterone is neuroprotective in lesioned or diseased nervous systems. Progesterone also facilitates the healing process after an injury. Females fare much better than males in the amount of brain damage that occurs after trauma, primarily because women have much higher levels of progesterone.[12]

Another important issue in MS is progesterone's ability to reduce lipid peroxidation, which produces free radicals—very unstable molecules that wreak havoc on our bodies. Levels of lipid peroxidation are much higher in people with MS.[13] Aging animals that have been treated

Lynne's Story

A 52-year-old attorney, Lynne received her MS diagnosis at age 47. Progressive weakness of her arm and leg began at 45. Her other symptoms included balance and coordination problems; arthritis; joint and muscle pain, stiffness, and cramping; tinnitus; bowel and bladder problems; chronic fatigue; emotional problems including anxiety and irritability; difficulty swallowing; cognitive problems; tremor; sleeping difficulties; neuralgia; carpal tunnel syndrome; and breathing difficulties. Her job became increasingly hard to do. Her memory was getting bad, and with her cognitive abilities also starting to worsen, she realized that she could not continue to work much longer.

Since the time of her diagnosis, Lynne also had been going through perimenopause. When her periods finally stopped, hot flashes, worse problems with sleep, and extreme irritability ensued. Shortly after this, her walking and balance became even more compromised and she had to start using a cane; her cognitive abilities also got worse. At her last visit, her neurologist told her that she would need to start thinking about making necessary changes to her house to accommodate a wheelchair.

This conversation finally spurred her into seeing another doctor, who friends had told her was having success treating symptoms of menopause—particularly brain fog. She didn't think she could handle having to stop work and going into a wheelchair at the same time.

> Her new doctor said the first order of business was to test her hormone levels. He also told her that he didn't want to get her hopes up but that he'd had some success in resolving not only menopause symptoms but also those of neurodegeneration with hormone treatment. Lynne's lab tests indicated low levels of estrogen, progesterone, testosterone, cortisol, and thyroid hormones. Lynne was put on bio-identical versions of all these hormones. Within several months, she was able to give up her cane and now has no balance or coordination issues at all. Hearing and breathing problems, and even the pain and numbness in her hands, are all resolved. Her mind is completely back to normal and her fear of having to stop working is gone—as is her likelihood of being in a wheelchair anytime soon!

with low doses of progesterone, estrogen, or a combination of both had reduced lipid peroxidation and less resulting damage.[14]

In summary, estrogen and progesterone play important roles in nerve health. Progesterone increases nerve connections, and both hormones stimulate formation of myelin sheaths.[15] Studies have also demonstrated that progesterone has neuroprotective consequences on the brain and spinal cord and promotes myelination in the central and peripheral nervous systems. Many studies have demonstrated that supplemental progesterone stimulates thickening of myelin sheaths and increases the rate of myelin formation.[16]

Why Do Progesterone Levels Drop Too Low?

Progesterone levels start to drop in women as early as their 30s and 40s (and even sometimes in their 20s). The most common reason for this is decreasing regularity of ovulation. If you remember that ovulation is necessary to release an egg and that the sac that surrounded the egg produces progesterone once the egg has left, then you can understand the traumatic effect on your body when this cycle doesn't occur. Because women continue to have periods without ovulation as long as they are still making some estrogen, they generally don't even know this is happening—this is truly "the silent killer." The only way to figure out what's going on is to have a blood test to measure your progesterone levels on days 19 to 22 of your menstrual cycle or test for ovulation with an ovulation test kit available at any drugstore.

Decreased progesterone production can stem from many things, including:

• Insufficient stimulation from the hypothalamus, pituitary, or

thyroid because of a problem with one of these glands
- Luteal phase defect, which simply means that you have ovulated but it hasn't resulted in adequate progesterone production in the luteal phase, or second half of your cycle. This results in infertility because adequate progesterone is necessary to ready the uterus to receive an egg.
- High cortisol (see Chapter 6 for more on this)
- High prolactin levels (see Chapter 7 for more on this)
- Antidepressant use
- Dietary—excessive sugar or saturated fat intake
- Deficiencies of vitamins A, B6, and C, and zinc
- Environmental exposure to many synthetic chemicals disrupts hormonal activity. They are called xenoestrogens because they have estrogen-like chemical structures that affect estrogen receptors. The resulting estrogenic exposure has been implicated in some extremely worrisome developments, such as greatly increasing numbers of hormone-related cancers, a 50% drop in sperm counts since 1940, and precocious puberty in children, including the recent finding that girls are starting menstruation an average of two years earlier.[17] Research over the last 20 years has also found that progesterone levels have started to drop at earlier and earlier ages, affecting girls in their teens or 20s.

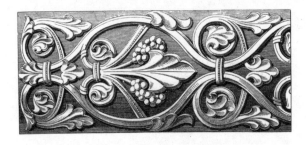

The Relationship Between Your Ovaries and Your Thyroid

The balance between estrogen and progesterone levels is important for another reason. Thyroid hormone and estrogen have opposing actions. When you don't ovulate and make enough balancing progesterone, the resulting excess estrogen competes with thyroid hormone and prevents it from binding to its receptor, so it never completes its mission. This causes hypothyroid symptoms even though you may have normal blood levels of thyroid hormone. It's important to detect and correct imbalances between estrogen and progesterone to prevent them from affecting your thyroid function.

Further, women's thyroids also have a mutually dependent relationship with estrogen and progesterone because our ovaries have receptors for thyroid hormone, and our thyroid has receptors for estrogen and progesterone. When estrogen and progesterone in women are low, it can cause decreased thyroid function. On the other hand, when thyroid function is low, it can cause lowered ovarian activity. This is why hypothyroidism is so common during perimenopause and menopause. These two conditions should be tested and treated together for optimal results.

Testosterone: Not Just for Men!

Although we immediately think of men when we hear the word "testosterone," it's critical to nerve health in women, as well. Ovaries produce half of our testosterone and the adrenals produce the other half. This setup sounds good because we can still hold out hope that we will have some testosterone left after our ovaries shut down at menopause, but most of us with MS have very little adrenal function left, so we are hit on both fronts.

Clinical studies show that testosterone plays a role in the inflammation, damage, and repair of nerves in MS. Women with multiple sclerosis have abnormally low testosterone levels, causing more disability, increased brain inflammation, and a greater number of gadolinium-enhancing lesions on MRIs (one of the current tests for MS). However, brain tissue damage also occurred in women with abnormally high levels of testosterone, so too much or too little appears to be a bad thing.[18]

Although men produce 20 to 30 times more testosterone than women do, it also plays a key role in women's physical and psychological health.[19] It's particularly important in sex drive and function of the sexual organs; building and maintaining muscle mass, fat, and energy; weight control; and sense of well-being. It has also been found important in preventing osteoporosis. By age 40, levels of testosterone drop to half of what they were at 20 and usually continue dropping.

On the other hand, some women end up with too much testosterone relative to remaining estrogen levels, which also causes problems as women find themselves with distressing symptoms such as excess hair growth, body fat redistribution, male-pattern baldness, acne, a deeper voice, increased muscle mass, an enlarged clitoris, increased sweating, and, more important, risk of MS disease progression.

Replacing Deficient Estrogen, Progesterone, and Testosterone

The best way to treat hormone deficiencies is to replace low hormones with ones that have the exact same molecular structure as those our bodies make, in a way that most closely mimics the way the body produces them. This seems like it would be common sense, as these hormones have kept us young and healthy for most of our lives. Unfortunately, because U.S. patent law prevents companies from patenting naturally occurring molecules, without these patents to protect their drugs from competition, few drug companies are willing to spend the money for FDA approval to make drug products out of them. Understanding this financial motivation is important. Doctors are only human, and because of their busy schedules, they tend to get most of their information from drug sales reps. This reality makes them experts on all the pharmaceutical solutions that are being heavily marketed, but unfortunately not on therapies still outside the mainstream.

> *Unfortunately, because U.S. patent law prevents companies from patenting naturally occurring molecules, without these patents to protect their drugs from competition, few drug companies are willing to spend the money for FDA approval to make drug products out of them.*

Hormone replacement therapy and the Women's Health Initiative conundrum. Hormone replacement therapy (HRT) with estrogen and progesterone has been heavily scrutinized recently, thanks to the Women's Health Initiative (WHI) clinical study, conducted by the National Institutes of Health. This study looked at the effects of Premarin (estrogens derived from horse urine) and Provera (medroxyprogesterone, or MPA, a molecularly altered progesterone), neither of which are recognized as estrogen and progesterone by our bodies. This study found that when used in combination, these two drugs cause a slight increase in heart disease, stroke, blood clots, and breast cancer. The group that used only the horse estrogens without MPA had far fewer side effects, showing that the MPA was causing most of the risk. Studies using bio-identical estrogen and progesterone molecules suggest that many of the side effects in the WHI study were related to the chemical alteration of progesterone and estrogen.

Unfortunately, when the findings from the WHI were published, the media didn't clarify that the drugs used were hormone products, not the actual hormones we make in our bodies. This oversight threw the medical community into a panic and many doctors responded by taking patients off hormones until they could sort out what it meant, leaving women with mass confusion. The one positive outcome of this study is that it has given visibility to the fact that standard hormone replacement therapy uses hormones unnatural to the body that do have negative side effects.

Altering progesterone molecular structure: what a nightmare! The biggest problem for those of us with MS is the progesterone-like product, MPA, that's currently being used both for hormone replacement and in birth control pills. This product actually interferes with your body's normal production and utilization of progesterone. It competes for the progesterone receptor binding sites. It stays in your body much longer than naturally occurring progesterone and can remain on the receptor site for up to six months. It doesn't stimulate the receptor in the same way that natural progesterone does.[20] (It would be interesting to do a study to see how many of us with MS took birth control pills at some point; could there be a connection?)

MPA doesn't balance estrogen as effectively as progesterone and only appears to protect against cell proliferation and cancer in the uterus, not other areas of the body. It negates many of the positive effects that estrogen potentially has on the heart, breast tissue, nerves, and cholesterol levels.[21] Many researchers believe that the WHI showed an increase in heart disease, not because of the effects of estrogen, but because MPA caused vasoconstriction, an increase in LDL cholesterol levels, and a decrease in HDL cholesterol levels.

Optimal delivery methods: stay away from oral dosing. Hormones should be replaced in a manner as similar as possible to the way the body makes them, so estrogen, progesterone, and testosterone should never be taken orally. This was another problem with the WHI: The horse estrogen products were given orally, which can increase blood pressure, triglycerides, and estrone—the estrogen we make in our fat cells primarily after menopause, which has been linked to heart disease and other negative health effects. This oral dosing can also cause gallstones and elevated liver enzymes (indicating that it's damaging the liver), and decrease growth hormone production (see Chapter 7 for more on this).

The best way to deliver estrogen replacement is transdermally, which means through the skin. I have found that patch products achieve the most even and reliable hormone levels. The sophisticated technology of these clear skin patches allows the hormone to be delivered in a measured, consistent way.

Oral progesterone also causes problems. When you take anything orally, it must first pass through your liver for processing (called a first-pass effect). When it does this, it creates by-products, or substances called metabolites, which can have unwanted consequences on your body. Even more concerning is that the levels of progesterone when taken orally never get high enough to protect your endometrium from cancer risk.[22] Clinical studies show that even though it results in lower blood levels than oral delivery, vaginal administration of progesterone protects the endometrium, suggesting a "first-pass uterine effect."[23] Because the uterus is what we are targeting (not the liver), this is possibly the better delivery method.

Beware of compounded hormones. One last word of caution as you enter this new, and hopefully health-changing, world of bio-identical hormones. You might go to a doctor who has worked with hormones and thinks that compounded hormone products provide a good option. Compounding is an FDA loophole that allows pharmacies to actually make their own drugs from raw materials—kind of like the apothecary shops of old. This practice gives flexibility for individual dosing regimens, which sounds good, but the problem is that there are no efficacy controls on the raw materials used in making these products. They are shipped in from Mexico, China, and other parts of the globe, with the only requirement being that they pass tests certifying that they are indeed the chemicals they represent they are—progesterone, estrogen, etc. They are not tested for efficacy as FDA-approved drug products are. They are not tested for the effect they have on symptoms nor the levels of hormones they create in the blood, so there are huge disparities in levels of hormones they create in our bodies, and subsequently how we feel when we take them.

I called the suppliers of the raw material, whom I knew from past drug development projects, and learned that they had no way of judging the efficacy of the products they sold—and they had no obligation under FDA regulations to do so.

I learned this fact the hard way, as I started out on these products and would feel great one month and horrible the next on a new batch of hormones. I come from the biotech world, so I applied some basic drug formulation principles to the situation. By testing my levels of the different hormones monthly, I quantified that there was indeed a huge disparity. One month my estrogen blood level would be very high, and the next month it would be very low. I felt like I was on a roller coaster. I called the suppliers of the raw material, whom I knew from past drug development projects, and learned that they had no way of judging the efficacy of the products they sold—and they had no obligation under FDA regulations to do so. The pharmacists don't have the specialized equipment to test for efficacy and also have no legal obligation to do so.

This experience forced me to research the bio-identical hormone products pharmaceutical companies were manufacturing under FDA guidelines that ensure pristine quality. I found that there are many excellent products on the market (read on for specifics).

Estrogen Replacement
Both research and anecdotal evidence suggest that lower levels of estrogen can make women more susceptible to autoimmune activity, but higher levels (associated with pregnancy) are protective. Higher levels of estrogen reduce not only disease severity but also the number and size of inflammatory lesions in the central nervous system. It also causes a shift in T1/T2 balance (which we discussed in Chapter 2) that is protective and anti-inflammatory.[24]

However, there exists no definitive proof of what the best estrogen level is for any individual. You must work with your doctor to figure out the right level for you, based on what it takes to resolve symptoms. Some women who have had higher estrogen levels their whole lives may need higher levels to resolve symptoms. HRT pioneer Elizabeth Vliet, M.D., says that women need levels of at least 90 to 100 pg/ml (picograms per milliliter) to feel good, maintain brain function and cardiovascular health, and prevent bone loss.[25] These are women in relatively good health, so by the time we get the symptoms of MS, we may need slightly higher levels.

> *There exists no definitive proof of what the best estrogen level is for any individual. You must work with your doctor to figure out the right level for you, based on what it takes to resolve symptoms.*

To feel my best, I find that I need to keep my levels between 100 and 150 pg/ml in the first two weeks of the month and 150 to 200 during the last two weeks, when I also supplement progesterone. If you look at the chart at the beginning of this chapter, you will see that estrogen levels always rise higher in the last two weeks of the month, when we have higher levels of progesterone. This is easy to accomplish: You simply use an extra whole or half patch (depending on what strength patch you are using) during this time. If you don't, you will probably notice that some of your symptoms will come back, as the estrogen-to-progesterone ratio has shifted and your estrogen is too low. Again, my levels are just an example; you may need very different levels, so work with your doctor to optimize your dosing regimen so that you enjoy the whole month symptom free.

There are many FDA-approved patch and gel products on the market. Each one delivers a different level of estrogen. Because those of us with neurodegenerative disease often need higher levels of estrogen, you will most likely need the higher-strength products, which are 0.1 mg/day. These products result in an average estrogen level of 100 pg/ml per patch. Some of them are Climara, Vivelle-Dot, and Alora. The gel products result in lower levels, so you will have to adjust doses accordingly.

The same products result in different estrogen levels for each woman, so it is important to measure your level after you start therapy. I have to use two of the 0.1 mg Vivelle-Dot patches to get to 200 pg/ml, but I have seen some women get levels of 40 and some at 160 on just one patch, so testing levels is imperative. I also have to change the patches every three days instead of every three and a half, as the manufacturers recommend, or I start to get symptoms back on the fourth day. Many women I have observed have also found this to be the case. You will use the estrogen as you need it, so you can empty a patch of estrogen much more quickly than three days—showing that your dose is too low.

One lesson I have learned is that the patch will start to irritate your skin when it no longer has any active ingredient (estrogen) in it. So if you start to get skin irritation, don't assume you are having a reaction to the patch; it's far more likely that you are just at too low a dose, ran out of estrogen early, and need to change the patch. Studies show that most women with MS are somewhat deficient in estrogen, but it is obviously very important that you quantify this. You may not be low at all or you may only be too low in the first half (or maybe even just the first week) of your cycle. It is important to ensure adequate levels all month long to obtain the important neuroprotective benefits of estrogen.

Progesterone Replacement
It's important to use progesterone in a way that mimics the normal menstrual cycle. The body naturally only has high levels of progesterone for

half the cycle for a reason: Progesterone balances and effectively blocks estrogen, which is important for cancer protection and many other reasons. However, if you supplement progesterone every day, you block some estrogen all the time and you will not get full benefit of its effects. Cyclic use of progesterone two weeks out of the month results in continued periods. If you are postmenopausal and have stopped having periods, you may be reluctant to start again. We need to put things in perspective when we have a disease like MS; research shows that mimicking the body's natural production of estrogen and progesterone is very beneficial. This should far outweigh the inconvenience of ongoing periods.

If you are still having periods and you can't tell if you're ovulating or not, you should buy an ovulation test kit to make sure. They're available at any drugstore and are easy to use. You should also measure your blood level of progesterone in a cycle in which you have ovulated. A level over 5 ng/ml (nanograms per milliliter) indicates that you have most likely ovulated—although it's still fairly low. If you ovulate and you have a low level, talk to your doctor about supplementing progesterone (even though you are still making some). If you don't ovulate, or ovulate very infrequently, you should consider using progesterone every month to get the most neurological benefit. Progesterone replacement may interfere with conception, so talk to your doctor about this if you are planning to conceive.

As mentioned earlier, progesterone shouldn't be taken orally. The optimum delivery method is vaginal. There are currently two progesterone products approved by the FDA that can be used vaginally (although they are not approved for HRT use). The first is Prochieve, manufactured by Columbia Labs. It is in a time-release formulation that lasts two days. It provides a reasonable solution, but personally, the one thing I don't like is that it delivers the progesterone evenly throughout the day and night. Like all hormones, progesterone is on a circadian rhythm, being higher in the morning and decreasing over the course of the day. When I use it, I sometimes have a hard time sleeping, as the level is too high at night. I have found that Prometrium, made by Solvay Pharmaceuticals, works better for me. This is actually an oral product, although in Europe it's sold for vaginal use, as well. I use 200 mg per day first thing in the morning, which has been shown to give a blood level of 8.26 ± 4.09 ng/ml.[26] Work with your doctor in measuring your progesterone level to make sure you are getting high enough levels to protect your endometrium (and also cause all that myelination!).

One last point to remember is that adequate estrogen is necessary to make progesterone receptors. Without it, progesterone supplementation will not be effective. The exact estrogen level required is not known, but one study has shown it to be above 30 pg/ml.[27]

Testosterone Replacement
Because studies show that adequate levels of testosterone are important in resolving MS, you should consider replacing it if your levels are low. If, instead, your testosterone levels are too high when you measure them, you should talk to your doctor about supplementing estrogen to balance it. As with the relationship between estrogen and progesterone, you must also have adequate estrogen to use testosterone effectively. Further, studies have shown that replacing testosterone without replacing estrogen can increase your risk of heart disease.

Testosterone should also be replaced transdermally. Because the limited FDA-approved products on the market are all approved for men, the dosage has to be adjusted for women. You may have to resort to a compounded product to achieve the levels your doctor recommends. It's important not to get your levels too high. The most common side effects of too high testosterone are facial hair growth and acne, but we also know that it has a negative impact on MS.

What You Need to Know About Testing

Because sex hormones are produced in a cyclic fashion during your menstrual cycle, what day you measure them in your cycle is crucial. Look back to the chart at the beginning of this chapter and you will see this issue's importance. Levels should always be measured before starting any replacement therapy and also regularly while undergoing therapy to make sure they are in optimal, safe ranges. You should get your blood drawn first thing in the morning while fasting. See the chart in Appendix A for complete information on optimal levels of the following hormones.

Progesterone: You need to measure progesterone in the middle of the second half of your cycle, when it is at its peak between days 19 and 22. If you have ovulated, your progesterone level will most likely be over 5 ng/ml, usually closer to 20 or 25.

Estradiol: This is the primary estrogen your ovaries make. We also make estriol (mainly during pregnancy) and estrone (mainly after menopause). Your doctor may want to measure estrone, as well, but estradiol is the estrogen we are mainly concerned with. If you are game to test two times during the month, measure once between days 1 and 3 to determine your level during the time when estrogen is lowest, and again between days 19 and 22 (at the same time you measure your progesterone level), when estrogen is at its highest except during ovulation. If you can only measure once, measure when you test progesterone on days 19 to 22 to start.

Testosterone: Testosterone can be measured at any time during your cycle, so the easiest time is when you are also measuring estrogen and progesterone.

Follicle stimulating hormone (FSH): This hormone stimulates your ovaries to make more estrogen when your pituitary senses that levels are too low. It's an indicator that you're starting to run out of eggs, so it's helpful but should not take the place of an estradiol test.

Key Points

- Estrogen supplementation not only results in resolving symptoms of MS in women, it actually *gets rid of* inflammatory lesions in the central nervous system.
- Progesterone has been shown to regenerate nerves and stimulate remyelination after lesions have occurred. It should be replaced in a cyclic fashion, two weeks out of every menstrual cycle, mimicking the body's natural production. This will result in continuing periods.
- Clinical studies show that testosterone plays an active role in MS. Levels too high or too low are associated with greater disability and numbers of brain lesions. Testosterone levels should be measured and replaced if low.
- Replacing sex hormones at the higher levels of youth or pregnancy has been shown to ameliorate symptoms of MS.
- It's important to use only bio-identical hormones to address deficiencies and imbalances. These are the same molecules that our bodies make and know just what to do with.

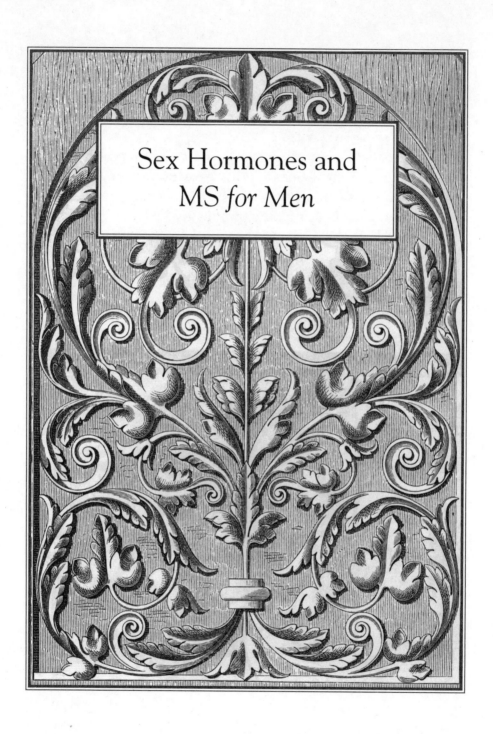

Sex Hormones and MS *for Men*

IV

The Importance of Testosterone

Sex hormones, including testosterone, estrogen, and progesterone, are just as important to men with MS as they are to women. When most men think of testosterone, the obvious thought of sex comes to mind—but testosterone is much more than just a "sex" hormone. All men have testosterone receptors throughout their body, not just the ones in their pelvic area. These receptors are also located in the brain, heart, and bones, to name a few. Testosterone is vital to almost every tissue and cell in a man's body. It's important in maintaining neurological and immune function, a healthy heart, and cholesterol levels; retaining muscle mass; forming new bone; making red blood cells; controlling blood sugar; and ensuring oxygenation in the entire body.

When men reach their 40s, they start to notice changes in their physical, sexual, and cognitive abilities. Outwardly, we start to see the hallmarks of the typical middle-aged male: increased abdominal fat, shrinking muscle mass, balding heads, and failing vision. Inwardly, even though most men don't like to admit it—and heaven forbid they should go to the doctor—they are starting to lose their sense of well-being, maybe even feeling depressed. This midlife depression often translates into feelings of worthlessness, lack of interest in activities that used to give them pleasure (you guessed it—this includes sex), anger, and irritability. They are having a hard time sleeping, they are starting to snore, their cholesterol is climbing, prostate problems are beginning, and energy levels are plummeting, leaving nighttime TV as the only viable entertainment.

Most men still believe these changes are just part of growing older, that they have to accept it. This common scenario tells the whole story: A sports fanatic has to transition from baseball to softball, then to over-40 softball, and finally stops entirely by 45 because the injury rate for jocks over this age is prohibitive. But should men have to settle for this? A remarkable amount of research has shown that the conditions and diseases that men begin to experience at middle age are caused by hormone imbalances and deficiencies, such as low testosterone levels—and that supplementing deficient hormones and supporting hormonal activity through good nutrition and lifestyle choices can correct these conditions.

> A remarkable amount of research has shown that the conditions and diseases that men begin to experience at middle age are caused by hormone imbalances and deficiencies, such as low testosterone levels—and that supplementing deficient hormones and supporting hormonal activity through good nutrition and lifestyle choices can correct these conditions.

Why Testosterone Levels Decline

Most men go through a change of life just as women do at menopause, except in men, it is called andropause. What are the symptoms of andropause? Fatigue, loss of energy, depression, irritability, anger, anxiety and stress, nervousness, memory loss and compromised concentration, decrease in job performance, diminished sex drive, loss of erections, lessened intensity of orgasms, backache and joint aches, loss of fitness, decline of physical abilities, bone loss, and elevated cholesterol levels.

Several things cause testosterone levels to drop more than they should. Testosterone production begins in the brain, in a gland called the hypothalamus. When it detects a deficiency of testosterone in the blood, it tells another gland, the pituitary, to ramp up production. The pituitary then tells cells in the testicles to produce more testosterone. Any injury to the brain—for men this often comes in the form of sports-related concussions—can affect the ability of your hypothalamus or pituitary to send the right signals. Other times, the problem lies with the testicles themselves. Some men's testicles lose their ability to respond to this command to produce more testosterone. But the end result is the same: not enough testosterone. Blood testing can determine where the problem originates—an important fact to establish, as the treatment differs depending on where the problem lies.

What Do the Women Say?

Results of a recent nationwide survey show that, sadly, more than half the women whose male partners have symptoms of low testosterone incorrectly think they are just part of the normal course of aging. The survey also found that women believe the symptoms of low testosterone negatively impact their relationship, and treatment with supplemental testosterone resulted in improving their relationship. The women surveyed said the symptoms of low testosterone included lack of energy (64%), decreased libido (61%), less strong erections (64%), a sad and/or grumpy mood (58%), and irritability (60%).[1]

Testosterone's Role in Inflammation and MS

One of testosterone's most important jobs is to control inflammation. We learned earlier of the damaging effects inflammation can have on the brain and how important an element it is in MS. Testosterone prevents detrimental cytokine production, which turns on C-reactive protein (a protein found in the blood), which goes up with inflammation, making this protein a good predictor of inflammatory conditions such as heart disease. So not only does testosterone work to resolve neurodegeneration, it is also good for your heart.[2] Testosterone has also been proven to shift our immune system to T2 dominance, which resolves inflammation.

> *Surprisingly, studies show that total testosterone in men with MS usually falls within the "normal" range, with it being low in only 24% of the men studied, so testosterone does not appear to be the only culprit.*

The obvious conclusion we draw on hearing how important testosterone is in resolving inflammation, as well as in nerve and immune function, is that men with MS must have low levels of testosterone. This thinking is what has probably thrown many researchers and doctors off the right track for so long. Surprisingly, studies show that total testosterone in men with MS usually falls within the "normal" range, with it being low in only 24% of the men studied, so testosterone does not appear to be the only culprit.[3] Of course, this takes us to the argument about what a "normal" range is; is it the testosterone level of an 80-year-old? I have seen 80-year-old men with testosterone ranges many times higher than a 40-year-old with MS who is theoretically in the normal range.

Further, most doctors don't look at free testosterone levels, which show how much testosterone is actually available to the body. You may have a decent amount of testosterone floating around in your blood, but much of it could be bound up by binding proteins, which make it unavailable for your body to use. The most significant hormone imbalance in aging men is this decrease in free testosterone, while at the same time estrogen levels remain the same or, in MS, increase dramatically. So the bottom line is that it is the balance between testosterone and estrogen in men that is most important. High estrogen causes your body to produce sex hormone binding globulin (SHBG), which binds testosterone in the blood and makes it unusable to your body. But let's put this aside and just agree for the moment that low testosterone may not be the primary problem for men with MS. If it isn't, what is?

The bottom line is that it is the balance between testosterone and estrogen in men that is most important.

Estrogen: Can't Live With It, Can't Live Without It

Clinical studies have proven that elevated estrogen is the real villain in MS, not low testosterone. Levels of estrogen in men with MS are four times higher than in healthy men, and the higher the estrogen levels, the greater the disability level and amount of tissue damage on an MRI.[4] But, virtually no doctor measures estrogen levels in men. Although estrogen is considered "the female hormone," the fact is that 60-year-old men have five times the estrogen of 60-year-old women. This is why as we age, we start to see women looking more like men, losing their hourglass shape and their hair, and men looking more like women,

Levels of estrogen in men with MS are four times higher than in healthy men, and the higher the estrogen levels, the greater the disability level and amount of tissue damage on an MRI.

with shrinking muscle mass and fat developing around the abdomen, hips, and breasts.

Men make estrogen from their testosterone. It's converted from testosterone with the help of an enzyme called aromatase. There is a lot of aromatase enzyme in fat cells, so overweight men usually have higher levels of estrogen. Men have important estrogen-sensitive tissues throughout the body, so they need to have enough estrogen for things like brain and sexual function. But the estrogen range for optimum performance is pretty narrow, so too much or too little will cause all kinds of problems.

In MS, the primary issue is inflammation, which testosterone is vital in controlling. Low testosterone causes a complex cascade of hormonal effects: When testosterone drops, it lowers growth hormone production, which results in more fat and more aromatase activity and—you got it—more estrogen. It also decreases insulin sensitivity, which triggers a condition called insulin resistance, another factor that increases fat cell mass. In insulin resistance, your body becomes insensitive to insulin after it has been doused with too high levels for too long (usually from eating too many simple carbs). Another dangerous effect of excess estrogen is an increased risk of stroke or heart attack and, the scourge of countless aging men, a swollen prostate.

Another strange biological quirk is that high levels of estrogen can trick your brain into thinking you are producing enough testosterone, which can further decrease your natural production. Estrogen stimulates testosterone receptors in your hypothalamus, which then stops telling your pituitary gland to stimulate your gonads to produce more testosterone; the entire feedback loop short-circuits. And, to further compound this problem, when you have too much estrogen, it attaches to testosterone receptor sites throughout your body and blocks the ability of your testosterone to use them, effectively blocking testosterone's action.

It doesn't matter how much testosterone (total or free) you have if excess estrogen is blocking your testosterone receptors.

Causes of High Estrogen Levels

Excess Aromatase Enzyme
As men age, they produce larger quantities of an enzyme called aromatase, which converts testosterone into estrogen in the body.

Obesity
Fat cells make aromatase, which creates more fat (especially abdominal fat), initiating a vicious cycle that makes even more fat. Low testosterone exacerbates this problem and causes even more aromatase production, which results in yet lower levels of testosterone and higher levels of estrogen.

Zinc Deficiency
As well as being important in overall pituitary function, zinc naturally inhibits the aromatase enzyme. When you are deficient in zinc, your estrogen levels may creep up.

Hypothyroidism
Low thyroid function causes impaired liver function, preventing your body from getting rid of estrogen effectively.

Lifestyle
Lifestyle choices such as drinking too much alcohol or eating too many refined carbs result in excess estrogen production. Excess alcohol also causes liver damage, which results in your body being unable to rid itself of excess estrogen.

Where Does Excess Estrogen Come From?

Okay, now that we know that excess estrogen is a major factor in MS, as well as in many other degenerative and inflammatory conditions, we need to look at what causes all this estrogen production. We discussed earlier that excess aromatase activity is a primary cause of high estrogen and is related to aging and too much fat. It is also caused by use of certain drugs, including diuretics (for high blood pressure), antifungal drugs, anticonvulsant drugs, high-dose glucocorticoids (Medrol and the like), antipsychotic drugs, statin drugs, and calcium channel blockers, just to name a few; decreased liver function; too much alcohol; zinc deficiency; and exposure to environmental estrogenic substances, such as fertilizers and pesticides.

What to Do to Reduce Estrogen

Because of the many damaging effects of excess estrogen, if you have MS it's important to measure your estrogen levels and reduce them if they're elevated. Here are some steps that you can take immediately to start to correct this problem.

If your estrogen level tests high (above 30 pg/ml, picograms per milliliter), you should consider the following actions to lower it:
- Reduce or eliminate alcohol consumption.
- Lose weight. Fat cells, especially those in the abdomen, make aromatase.
- Take 80 to 100 mg per day of zinc.
- Take 600 mg per day of a saw palmetto and beta-sitosterol combination. It may reduce the effects of excess estrogen by blocking the estrogen receptor sites in prostate cells.
- Take 240 mg a day of nettle extract (*Urtica dioica*). Nettle can inhibit SHBG, which, in turn, makes more of your testosterone available to your body.

- Take 400 mg of indole-3-carbinol to help neutralize estrogen. This is made of cruciferous vegetables such as broccoli and cauliflower and can help your liver to metabolize and excrete excess estrogen. It can be purchased at most health food stores or online (as can the other supplements mentioned previously).
- Take 100 mg of supplemental bio-identical progesterone, which reduces estrogen levels by approximately 35%.[5]
- With your doctor, review all drugs you are taking to see if they may be interfering with your liver function. Common drugs that affect liver function are NSAIDs such as ibuprofen, acetaminophen, and aspirin; the statin class of cholesterol-lowering drugs; some heart and blood-pressure medications; and some antidepressants.
- The last resort is a prescription drug called Arimidex (anastrozole), as it has some nasty side effects. If all else fails, talk to your doctor about this option.

The Relationship Between Testosterone and Thyroid

Men's thyroids have a mutually dependent relationship with their testicles because testicles have receptors for thyroid hormone, and their thyroid has receptors for testosterone. When testosterone is low, it can cause decreased thyroid function. On the other hand, when thyroid function is low, it can cause lowered testicular activity. This is why hypothyroidism becomes more common during andropause. Levels of both testosterone and thyroid hormones should always be measured and treated together.

Why Is Progesterone Important?

Progesterone is the body's natural balance for estrogen. Women make very high levels of progesterone in their ovaries and men make a relatively small amount in their testicles and adrenal glands. Surprisingly, given its virtual lack of use in the treatment of MS, a large amount of research data is available showing progesterone's vital role in myelination and remyelination. It both preserves and restores the integrity of myelin sheaths and enables fast and efficient conduction of electrical impulses along nerve fibers. Progesterone has been shown to actually regenerate nerves after lesions have occurred.[6] It's thought to protect and regenerate nerves by accelerating the formation of new myelin sheaths, and by acting directly on your neurons to increase survival.[7] Read the section in Chapter 3 titled "Progesterone's Role in MS" to learn more about this hormone's effect on myelination and remyelination.

Surprisingly, given its virtual lack of use in the treatment of MS, a large amount of research data is available showing progesterone's vital role in myelination and remyelination.

When men have too much estrogen and not enough progesterone, their blood vessels become lumpy, which makes them prone to clotting diseases such as stroke and angina. Progesterone is important in allowing the vessels to relax properly. It's safe to say that progesterone is necessary to maintain cardiovascular health.

Without adequate progesterone, men also tend to get osteoporosis, just like women. For more on this hormone, see the following list of progesterone's functions for men.

Functions of Progesterone in Men

Progesterone serves many of the same important purposes in men as in women:

- Critical for nerve health and causes remyelination
- Important in memory and cognitive function
- Stimulates bone growth and helps prevent osteoporosis
- Protects your heart by maintaining vascular tone and optimal cholesterol levels
- Helps prevent blood clots and guards against stroke
- Ensures optimal immune function
- Necessary for sex drive and function
- Normalizes sleep
- Ensures bladder health
- Balances estrogen-induced cell proliferation
- Affects mood—has calming effect on brain neurons
- Critical to effective adrenal and thyroid function
- Sensitizes estrogen receptors
- Maintains blood sugar control
- Is a precursor, or building block, for other hormones
- Facilitates healing process after an injury. Females fare much better than males in the amount of brain damage that occurs after cerebral strokes, primarily because females have much higher levels of progesterone.[8]
- Adequate progesterone results in less water retention in the brain. For this reason, some neurosurgeons use progesterone injections before surgery to prevent swelling due to water retention.

Why Do Progesterone Levels Drop?

When you see how crucial progesterone is to your health in so many ways, you realize why it's important to make sure you have enough of it. The following are some reasons why it can drop and lead to health problems; again, many are the same in men and in women:

- Insufficient stimulation from the hypothalamus, pituitary, or thyroid because of a problem with one of these glands
- High cortisol (see Chapter 6 for more on this)
- High prolactin levels (see Chapter 7 for more on this)
- Antidepressant use
- Dietary—excessive sugar or saturated fat intake
- Deficiencies of vitamins A, B6, and C and zinc
- Environmental exposure to many synthetic chemicals introduced in the last 50 years disrupts hormonal activity. These chemicals are called xenoestrogens because they have estrogen-like chemical structures that interfere with estrogen receptors, creating an estrogen-like effect on the body. The resulting estrogenic exposure has been implicated in some extremely worrisome health trends, such as the increase in hormone-related cancers and precocious puberty in children, as well as a 50% drop in sperm counts since 1940.[9]

Estrogenic exposure has been implicated in some extremely worrisome health trends, such as the increase in hormone-related cancers and precocious puberty in children, as well as a 50% drop in sperm counts since 1940.

Mike's Story

Mike, 46, was diagnosed with MS at age 42. His primary symptoms were severe pain in his legs and feet, depression, and balance problems. He didn't have cognitive or memory problems, but his libido and ability to achieve and maintain erections were affected. Along with his balance problems, his right leg had gotten very numb, making walking harder and harder. His right hand was also affected to a lesser degree; its slight numbness made tasks such as buttoning up buttons and picking up small objects difficult.

As in many men, Mike's MS was progressing fairly rapidly. In four short years, his ability to walk was noticeably diminished. A measurement of Mike's hormone levels revealed that his testosterone was in the mid-200s, very low for his age, and his estrogen level was at 58, much too high. His growth hormone level was also quite low, as was his DHEA (an adrenal hormone) level. His progesterone, too, fell under the normal range.

Mike's doctor decided to start him on a testosterone patch to increase his testosterone levels and a dose of human growth hormone (HGH) to bring him into its optimal range. He also started him on 100 mg of progesterone to bring his levels up to enhance myelination of his nerves, as well as balance and lower his estrogen levels. He added doses of zinc, saw palmetto with beta-sitosterol, and indole-3-carbinol to further lower his estrogen levels. Also, Mike's level of magnesium was very low, so his doctor gave him 1,200 mg per day to address this deficiency; he had him take 300 mg in the morning, 300 at noon, and 600 at night because Mike's stiffness and pain were worse at night and first thing in the morning.

Mike's thyroid tests were not conclusive. His TSH and T4 thyroid hormones fell in normal ranges, but his T3 was in the low end of the range. Given the fact that many people with MS have disproportionately low levels of T3, the body's most active thyroid hormone, Mike's doctor decided to supplement this as well with a combination T3 and T4 thyroid product. He started him at 60 mg of Armour thyroid, with a plan to increase his dose steadily until his symptoms resolved.

Mike noticed a huge difference the first day he started on these therapies. On a scale of 1 to 10, his pain went from a 9 to a 5. He could get out of bed the first morning without cramping up so badly that it took half an hour to start walking, which is what he had become used to during the past several years. The muscle spasms that kept him awake at night resolved with the 1,200 mg of magnesium. Mike's doctor slowly increased his dose of Armour thyroid until he reached 120 mg. The pain and stiffness that had started to resolve almost immediately disappeared with the 120 mg dose. The combination of progesterone, zinc, saw palmetto with beta-sitosterol, and indole-3-carbinol successfully lowered his estrogen level to 32. Combined with his testosterone level, which had climbed to 740, this decreased estrogen level had Mike fully functional sexually again. The last time Mike saw his doctor, he told him, "I don't even feel like I have MS anymore!"

Treatment Options

Testosterone Replacement

Depending on your test results, your doctor may decide to treat you with testosterone or something called human chorionic gonadatropin hormone (HCG). HCG is very similar to the luteinizing hormone made in the pituitary, which signals your testes to make testosterone. It will be used if your low testosterone is caused by a malfunction on the part of your pituitary or hypothalamus. Using it two to three times a week by injection can jump-start the testes into resuming production.

If the trouble lies with your testes, testosterone will be given. Testosterone should be administered transdermally by skin patch, time-release gel, or cream, or by an implantable pellet. Do not use testosterone injections or oral tablets. Both oral testosterone and injections raise testosterone levels too high, and then they drop too quickly. This doesn't make you feel good, and it can also raise estrogen above desired levels. Oral testosterone also raises "bad" cholesterol and lowers the "good" kind. And, if that's not enough, it's banned in all modernized countries except Canada and the United States. Transdermal delivery of testosterone is much more effective for erectile dysfunction. It works 81% of the time, compared with just 53% for intramuscular administration and 51% when given orally.[10] There are several types of transdermal products available, including skin patches and gel, that are FDA approved. They are very good quality; if you can afford them, they are the best way to go. Compounded drugs are cheaper but have significant drawbacks. See "Beware of Compounded Hormones" in Chapter 3 for an important word of caution.

Free and total testosterone blood levels should be in the upper end of the reference range for men 21 to 29 years old. Labs have different ranges for different ages, but to ameliorate symptoms of MS, anecdotal evidence shows that levels should be slightly higher than in healthy men. The reference range from Quest Diagnostics Lab for total testosterone is 250 to 1,100 ng/dl (nanograms per deciliter). This means your target will be somewhere between 600 and 1,100 ng/dl. Work with your doctor to find the right dose to achieve levels that resolve your symptoms; this level is different for each person. Individual responses to the same dose of testosterone also vary, so it's important to measure blood levels when you start supplementing.

Progesterone Replacement
Your progesterone level should be at least 1.2 ng/ml (nanograms per milliliter) for optimal neurological protection. Consider using progesterone suppositories, if possible, particularly if you have benign prostate hypertrophy, because they will reduce local levels of estrogen in the prostate. Take 25 to 100 mg every morning in either suppository or transdermal cream form. If you take it orally (which is not optimal, as it causes metabolites when processed through your liver), it should be taken at night because it causes drowsiness. Always measure blood levels after you begin supplementation to make sure optimal levels are being achieved.

What You Need to Know About Testing

The following are the basic blood tests to start with. You should get your blood drawn first thing in the morning while fasting. See the chart in Appendix A for complete information on optimal levels of the following hormones.

Testosterone: Have total and free levels measured. The free levels are the amount of hormone that's biologically active in your body—rather than total levels. When testosterone reaches target levels, you should monitor blood levels of estradiol, free and total testosterone, and PSA approximately every 45 days for the first six months and then work with your doctor to continue to check levels regularly.

Estrogen: Measuring estrogen levels is always important when you supplement testosterone because it can convert to even more estrogen in your body. There are several different types of estrogen. Estradiol is the type that should be tested. The objective is to raise your levels of total and free testosterone but keep your estradiol levels under 30 pg/ml. This should be retested when you retest testosterone. Your doctor may also want to measure estrone, which is a type of estrogen that is made primarily in fat cells; so the more fat you have, the more estrone you make. It can lead to prostate enlargement, heart disease, and weight gain.

Progesterone: This is a key hormone for those with MS, as it has been proven critical in remyelination of the nerves. Progesterone should be tested initially and then retested when you retest testosterone and estrogen.

PSA: PSA stands for prostate-specific antigen, which is a protein that indicates activity in the prostate gland; the higher it is, the more activity. You should have a baseline PSA blood test and a digital rectal exam to check for prostate cancer before you consider testosterone replacement, and then every 30 to 45 days for the first six months. Conventional doctors are concerned that testosterone replacement therapy causes prostate cancer. This has not been scientifically validated and research suggests that when testosterone levels decrease, prostate cancer increases.[11] But if you have existing cancer, most doctors will not be comfortable with testosterone replacement because it might exacerbate it. Until this issue has been medically proven, it's best to err on the side of caution.

> *Conventional doctors are concerned that testosterone replacement therapy causes prostate cancer. This has not been scientifically validated and research suggests that when testosterone levels decrease, prostate cancer increases.*

SHBG: Sex hormone binding globulin is a protein that binds testosterone so that it isn't available to your cells. It increases normally with age but also with higher estrogen levels. SHBG should be under 40 pmol/l (picomoles per liter).

LH (luteinizing hormone) and FSH (follicle stimulating hormone): These two hormones made by your pituitary tell you if low testosterone is caused by a problem with the pituitary or with your testes. If your testosterone levels are low and these two levels are also low, then this result indicates a problem with your pituitary because it should be making more LH and FSH to stimulate testosterone production. If they are high and testosterone is low, then the problem is with your testes because they aren't responding properly to the message being sent by your pituitary. The optimal level for LH is 3 mIU/ml (million international units per milliliter); (over 8 is too high). For FSH, 2 mIU/ml is optimal, and over 7 is too high.[12]

Key Points

- Clinical studies show that elevated estrogen is common in men with MS and is possibly the cause of damaging inflammation.
- You should have your estrogen levels measured and follow the suggestions for lowering levels if they are above 30 pg/ml.
- Testosterone is critical to nerve health. Both free and total testosterone should be measured, as well as sex hormone binding globulin, to make sure that you have enough testosterone available to your cells.
- Testosterone should be administered transdermally by skin patch, time-release gel or cream, or by an implantable pellet. Do not use testosterone injections or oral tablets as they raise testosterone levels too high, and then they drop too quickly.
- Progesterone is also important to men in maintaining healthy nerve function as well as balancing estrogen. Levels should be measured and replaced if low.
- Take progesterone every morning in either suppository or transdermal cream form. Consider using progesterone suppositories, if possible, particularly if you have benign prostate hypertrophy, because they will reduce local levels of estrogen in the prostate. If you take it orally (which is not optimal, as it causes metabolites when processed through your liver), it should be taken at night because it causes drowsiness.
- All hormone levels should be tested prior to initiating hormone therapy and regularly thereafter to monitor levels.

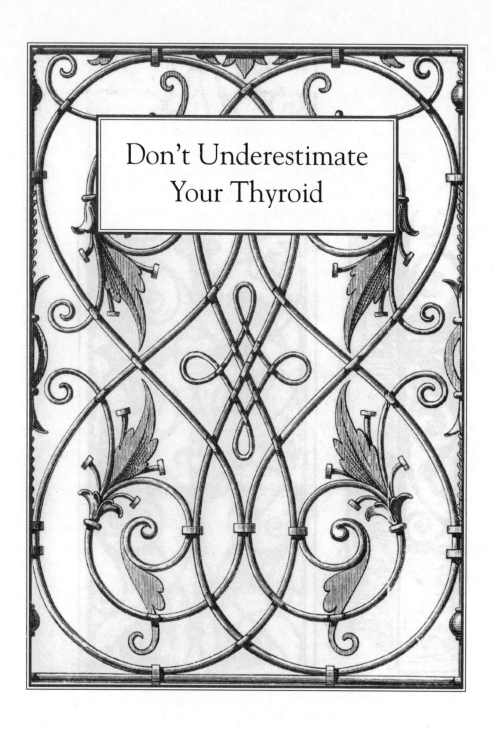

Don't Underestimate Your Thyroid

V

The Importance of Your Thyroid

Initially, it's difficult to grasp just how important your thyroid can be in MS. Most of us have never even heard of it, let alone realize it might have something to do with our condition. I'm willing to bet that none of the many doctors you have seen in your quest to find out what's wrong even mentioned it. Yet, thyroid function is one of the first things that should be investigated when someone starts showing signs of neurological malfunction.

Why? Your thyroid gland is your first line of defense against threats from the outside world. It's one of the most important glands in detoxifying and neutralizing viruses and bacteria, as well as harmful things you eat, drink, or breathe. We even make our own toxic substances when our food decomposes, as well as during the process of metabolism in our tissues. The bottom line is that, along with other glands and organs, the thyroid destroys and eliminates all these poisonous materials from your body. When these glands are working as they should, we can withstand massive assaults from our environment. But, when the thyroid isn't doing its job, we can't get rid of this toxic burden, and it's not surprising we get sick.

Second, and just as important, the thyroid serves as the engine for your metabolism. This doesn't sound all that interesting until you realize that metabolism simply means the process of turning food into energy. When your metabolism isn't working at full speed, everything in your body slows down: Every organ, gland, even cell, is affected. Is it any wonder that when we have low thyroid function we start slowly, insidiously deteriorating? A general slowing of all physical and mental processes occurs. It reduces oxygen consumption, slowing down utilization of nutrients for energy. Our skin gets dry and our extremities get cold. We can't regulate our body temperature. (Are you always cold? How long has it been since you actually sweated?) We're often constipated and are always tired, and how can you expect your mind to work when it has no fuel?

> *Thyroid function is one of the first things that should be investigated when someone starts showing signs of neurological malfunction.*

Low thyroid function, or hypothyroidism, is a widespread and growing condition. Belgian endocrinologist Dr. Jacques Hertoghe estimated worldwide incidence to be as high as 80%![1] Other estimates say 25% of all women will develop hypothyroidism, with the greatest incidence occurring after age 34.[2] Women make up 80% of all cases of thyroid disease—closely mimicking the distribution of MS between men and women. And finally, studies have shown that thyroid disorders are at least three times more common in women with MS than in the general population.[3]

> *Low thyroid function, or hypothyroidism, is a widespread and growing condition.*

Always Look at Your Symptoms

Let's go back to our list of MS symptoms and see what part your thyroid may play in each of them. Other hormones can sometimes be involved in these symptoms, as well, but they are well-known symptoms of hypothyroidism. Most of them are thought to be caused by a common problem in hypothyroidism called myxedema. This condition results from the accumulation of waste products that aren't effectively excreted when hypothyroidism slows down metabolism. When this happens, a jellylike substance called mucin, located throughout our tissues, attracts water and swells up. This condition develops insidiously. It's often not physically obvious but collects internally around organs and glands, causing all kinds of problems. When it does become obvious, it most commonly can be seen in swelling around the eyes and the front of the upper arms and thighs. It almost feels as if the skin has thickened, as it's hard to pinch it between two fingers.

Studies have shown that thyroid disorders are at least three times more common in women with MS than in the general population.

Numbness and tingling: My first symptom was numbness and tingling in my hands. It started in my right hand and then spread to my left. The neurologist I went to said it was carpal tunnel syndrome, caused by compression of a nerve in my wrist, triggered by repetitive motion. I thought this diagnosis was peculiar because except for some computer work, I really did nothing that required repetitive motion of my hands. He said nothing could be done for it other than surgery, which he encouraged me to have. This is the problem I have found with most "-ologists," doctors who specialize in something—they look at specific body parts as if they were detached from the rest of the body.

In fact, one of the most common causes of carpal tunnel is low thyroid function. Low thyroid causes swelling in the connective tissues around the nerves; the pressure this swelling creates can cause tingling, numbness, and pain—in other words, carpal tunnel syndrome. The fact that women are three times more likely than men to develop it and that it has a peak incidence around age 42 should give us clues that it's hormonal in nature. Most conditions that have a greater incidence in women are hormone related.

Fatigue: When you realize that your thyroid runs your body's metabolism and actually fuels those little energy generators in every cell called mitochondria, it's obvious why low thyroid results in fatigue. Low metabolic function affects every cell in your body, kind of like running out of gas. When I started on the right dose of thyroid hormones, the change was dramatic. My fatigue lifted overnight.

Bladder and bowel: Your bowel and bladder also get caught up in the whole slowing process. Many of us with MS have chronic constipation. This isn't surprising because when we have low thyroid, it's like functioning in slow motion. Later in the progression, it's also common to get bowel incontinence.

I had numerous bladder problems. The urologist I went to said I had a common condition, something called a "lazy bladder," in which the bladder is full but can't void itself. I thought to myself, "My bladder is far from lazy!" It had me jumping out of bed many times a night with a feeling of urgency, burning, and pain (later diagnosed as something called interstitial cystitis). In MS, catheterization is often required to empty the bladder, and I had to make a couple of disheartening trips to the emergency room to have this done. I was starting to think I would have to learn to master the art of catheterization when I found the hormone connection. When I started on estrogen and progesterone, my bladder problems got significantly better, but adding thyroid and cortisol got rid of them entirely.

Balance problems and decreased coordination: Many people with MS have problems with coordination and balance. This can also be caused by hypothyroidism, in which the difficulties are thought to result from increased fluids building up in the part of the brain concerned with motor skills as well as the spinal nerves.[4] I was very unsteady on my feet for several years and my knees felt like they were going to give out if I started to walk fast or run (and actually did on occasion). Thyroid replacement resolved both of these problems.

Vision abnormalities: I lost most of the eyesight in my right eye, and my left eye was blurry much of the time (although, strangely enough, not all the time.) Thyroid and estrogen replacement restored my vision completely and I no longer even need reading glasses. Thyroid deficiency causes swelling in tissues as waste products build up, and the increased fluid this causes in the cornea is thought to be the source of vision problems. Low levels of estrogen in women and testosterone in men can also cause eyesight problems and have been linked to increases in dry eye syndrome, vision loss, macular degeneration, glaucoma, and cataracts.[5]

Cognitive impairment: Most of us with MS have experienced times when our cognitive abilities have been affected. In my observation, women seem to have more cognitive trouble than men do; this may be due to the basic biological differences between the brains of men and women. Women have fewer actual brain cells than men have, but they have far more connections to other parts of the brain for each of these cells, allowing them to use more areas of the brain at the same time. Because far larger areas of women's brains are used at a given time, they require more energy and increased blood flow to fuel cognitive tasks. Low thyroid hormone levels cause an actual decrease in brain function. Thyroid hormones, as well as estrogen in women and testosterone in men, ensure optimum blood flow.[6]

Sleep problems: Deep sleep is crucial to the repair of muscles and nerves. Hypothyroidism often causes insomnia, as do estrogen or progesterone deficiencies. Hypothyroidism usually results in having a hard time falling asleep, whereas with low estrogen for women or low testosterone for men, you can fall asleep but you sleep lightly and wake up often.

Emotional lability, mood swings, and depression: These symptoms are all common in hypothyroidism. There are many thyroid receptors in the brain, and when they are not being effectively stimulated, emotional and psychological problems are common. Many experts in thyroid function believe that thyroid tests should be performed on any patient with these symptoms, as well as anyone with psychoses, bipolar disorder, paranoia, or schizophrenia.[7] Unfortunately, many of us think we're just going crazy, instead of getting to the root of the problem and fixing our thyroid function.

> *Unfortunately, many of us think we're just going crazy, instead of getting to the root of the problem and fixing our thyroid function.*

Sexual dysfunction: This is very common in both sexes in MS. Thyroid is critical to libido and sexual performance (as are estrogen, testosterone, and progesterone).[8]

Muscle and joint stiffness and cramping: Muscle health depends on thyroid, and without adequate hormone levels, muscles can become sluggish and infiltrated with fat, which can cause pain, stiffness, and cramping.[9] Pain and cramping in hands, feet, and neck is specifically thyroid related.

Speech problems: Speech is also affected by low thyroid. When this happens, the voice can become deliberate and slow. Articulating words is difficult, and it's common to stumble over words and slur as if drunk. These difficulties can stem from swelling of the tongue and lips. The tongue sometimes looks scalloped and/or thick in this condition. The voice also often changes and can become hoarse and soft.

Pain: Also called arthralgia, pain is common in MS and hypothyroidism. This is caused by muscle fibers separating due to edema and reduced muscle enzyme activity caused by low metabolism.[10]

Other Signs and Symptoms of Hypothyroidism

There are many other symptoms of low thyroid that are not commonly considered "MS" symptoms, but many of us who have MS also have them. How many symptoms do you have? Put a check mark next to any you have experienced.

- __ Accelerated aging
- __ Anemia
- __ Anxiety
- __ Asthma
- __ Attention-deficit/hyperactivity disorder (ADHD)
- __ Back and/or leg pain
- __ Blood pressure abnormalities (high or low)
- __ Cervical dysplasia in women
- __ Chronic colds and illness
- __ Cognitive and memory problems
- __ Cold hands and feet
- __ Depression
- __ Difficulty swallowing
- __ Dry, coarse skin
- __ Dull or yellowish eyes
- __ Early onset of menopause or andropause
- __ Easy bruising
- __ Elevated cholesterol
- __ Enlarged abdomen
- __ Excess flatulence
- __ Fibrocystic breast disease
- __ Fibromyalgia
- __ Hair loss or thinning, or coarse, dry, or brittle hair on body and head
- __ Having a hard time breathing
- __ Headaches
- __ Hearing problems and/or tinnitus
- __ Heart enlargement seen on X-ray
- __ Heart palpitations
- __ Hemorrhoids
- __ Infertility
- __ Insomnia and sleep problems
- __ Intolerance of cold or heat
- __ Irritability
- __ Lack of appetite
- __ Lack of sweating
- __ Liver swelling or pain
- __ Low basal body temperature
- __ Muscle and joint stiffness, weakness, and/or pain
- __ Pain in the hands, feet, or neck
- __ Painful, heavy, or irregular periods in women
- __ Pale or bluish skin, nail beds, lips, or mucous membranes
- __ Premature graying of hair

___ Premenstrual syndrome
___ Puffy face and eyelids
___ Recurrent upper respiratory infections
___ Restless legs syndrome
___ Skin disorders such as eczema and psoriasis
___ Slow Achilles reflex
___ Sluggish movement
___ Strange thoughts and psychological problems
___ Swollen feet and legs
___ Thickening of the neck or development of a goiter
___ Thin, brittle, ridged fingernails
___ Thinning eyebrows, especially at the outer ends
___ Tingling in the hands and feet
___ Urinary tract infections
___ Vivid, disturbing dreams
___ Weak, slow, or soft pulse
___ Weight gain
___ Yeast infections

How Does Your Thyroid Work?

Looking at these lists of symptoms gives us an idea of how vital our thyroid function can be in MS. Because thyroid malfunction is pretty complex, to get to the bottom of what's going on in your personal situation, it's important to understand the basics of how your thyroid works. Your thyroid function involves an intricate interplay with several other glands, primarily your hypothalamus and pituitary. The hypothalamus regulates your endocrine system. It stimulates your pituitary to produce something called thyroid stimulating hormone (TSH), which then tells your thyroid to make more thyroid hormone if your levels are too low, or to slow production if they are too high. These glands continually monitor and adjust the amount of thyroid hormone to keep it within a narrow optimal range.

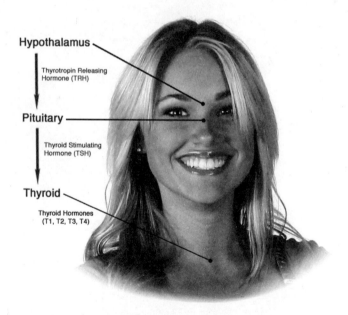

Thyroid Hormone Production Pathway

Your Thyroid Hormones

Your thyroid makes things happen via four thyroid hormones, commonly called T1, T2, T3, and T4. They're all necessary for your thyroid to accomplish its tasks. No one is quite sure yet what T1 does, although I'm hopeful that with all the attention researchers, the media, and the public are finally paying to the importance of thyroid function in health, it won't be long until we understand it completely. Scientists believe it may control the electrical input and charge of the brain in some way. T2 increases the metabolic rate of muscles and fat tissue.[11] But T3 and T4 do most of the work. T4, the most abundant thyroid hormone in the body, partially derives from iodine in your diet. It must be converted to T3 to have any effect on the body, as we have T3 hormone receptors but none for T4. This might seem like obscure and unnecessary information, but it's important when we get around to discussing what type of hormone should be used in thyroid therapy.

My Story

Understanding the complex interplay of thyroid hormones was critical in understanding and fixing my own health. Doctors currently evaluate thyroid status by measuring TSH and often total T4 levels. This practice makes some sense because TSH continues to rise as the levels of thyroid hormones decrease. Unfortunately, it tells us only a small part of the story. If something has gone awry with your hypothalamus or pituitary, your TSH will generally remain at normal levels but you may still have an inadequate amount of thyroid hormone to maintain good health. This is because some malfunction makes the hypothalamus or pituitary unable to respond effectively and increase TSH production as they should when thyroid levels drop. And even a slight increase or decrease in thyroid effect can alter the activity in your cells, wreaking havoc on your body. Measuring T4 is also important, but the free level is more valuable than the total level because this is what is actually available to your cells.

The initial thyroid tests I had were for TSH and T4. My levels were very low but still in "normal" ranges (T4 was 0.9 in a range of 0.71 to 1.85, and TSH was 0.95 in a range of 0.49 to 4.67). When I finally got around to having my level of T3 (the type of thyroid hormone that is most biologically active in our bodies) tested quite a while later, we found that it was almost nonexistent: 0.1 in a range of 2.3 to 6.6. Because this test is virtually never done, most doctors wouldn't have detected my thyroid problem—although, depressingly enough, no doctor ever thought to check any of my thyroid levels in treating my MS. It was clearly one of the reasons I had so many severe symptoms.

Very low TSH as well as low T3 and T4 showed a problem with my hypothalamus and/or pituitary function. This is called central hypothyroidism, and unfortunately most doctors don't know it exists so they never test for it.

Later, I found copies of some old labs that I had done when I first started to explore my numb hands 14 years ago. Strangely enough, the doctor had tested T3, T4, and TSH. My levels were almost identical to those measured 11 years later: very low T3, T4, and TSH, indicative of central hypothyroidism. Unfortunately, my doctor didn't pick up on this or I probably would have had a very different outcome if he had.

What Causes Hypothyroidism?

One of the challenges in getting to the bottom of what's going on is figuring out what went wrong in the first place. Lots of internal and external factors can affect your thyroid. Don't despair, though, if you don't have the resources to do extensive testing to find out exactly what caused your thyroid to malfunction. If your basic lab tests and/or symptoms convince your doctor that your thyroid might be an issue in your MS, a trial course of thyroid replacement will quickly show if it is the right path for you without having to test levels of such things as vitamins, minerals, and heavy metals. The following are some of the things that can cause thyroid problems.

> *One of the challenges in getting to the bottom of what's going on is figuring out what went wrong in the first place. Lots of internal and external factors can affect your thyroid.*

A Problem with Your Thyroid

Often something goes wrong with your thyroid itself, including:
- Direct or indirect physical trauma to the thyroid, such as surgery or whiplash
- Exposure to certain viruses
- Genetic inheritance
- Diet also plays an important role. Avoid eating a diet too low, or unbalanced, in protein, fat, or carbohydrates, as well as excessive amounts of cruciferous vegetables, alcohol, walnuts, or soy.
- Toxic environmental exposure including X-rays, chemicals (e.g., fluoride, heavy metals, pesticides, dioxins, and PCBs), and nuclear fallout (disasters such as Chernobyl and Three Mile Island spread nuclear fallout around the world)

- Long-term iodine deficiency
- Autoimmune disease or thyroid antibodies
- Medications that interfere with your thyroid function, including estrogen (when it's not properly balanced by progesterone), birth control pills, beta-blockers, lithium, phenytoin, theophylline, and chemotherapy

A Problem with Another Gland

Hypothyroidism may result from a problem with your hypothalamus or pituitary gland, which regulate the thyroid, and can be caused by many things, including head injuries, a growth on one of the glands, or genetic disorders.[12]

Inherited Problems

Inherited deficiencies can also cause low thyroid function. These can result from genetic issues that are too complex to go into here, and because the treatment is the same whether it's a genetic problem or not, it may not be worth the expense to test for this. I have tested for genetic problems and found that I, and the two of my three sons who I have had tested, possess the genetic markers for MS (something called HLA class II complex, in particular HLA-DR15Dw2 and DQw6).[13]

When a parent has the following conditions, be on the lookout for inherited low thyroid function in his or her offspring: excessive drinking, X-ray exposure, and, strangely enough, gout—as well as any of the other factors that damage the thyroid. Any type of insufficient parental thyroid function can be inherited. Children of alcoholics should be especially alert for signs of low thyroid function. Low thyroid function can cause a predisposition to alcoholism, so maybe some inherited drinking problems are really inherited low thyroid function (often combined with low adrenal function).[14]

Conversion Problems

A fourth problem is the inability to convert T4 to T3 effectively. Even if you have enough T4, you may not be able to convert it to T3 because many things can affect the enzyme responsible for this conversion, including deficiencies of selenium, iodine, iron, potassium, zinc, copper, and vitamins A, B, C, and E; stress; cadmium, mercury, and lead toxicity; starvation; inadequate or excessive protein intake; elevated cortisol; chronic illness; excessive alcohol consumption; and decreased kidney or liver function. Clinical studies have shown that many people with MS have much lower levels of T3 but fairly normal levels of T4. This makes it likely that many with MS have this low T3 syndrome caused by impaired T4-to-T3 conversion, possibly with increased T4 conversion to reverse T3.

What Is Reverse T3?

Reverse T3 is made when T4 is converted normally into both T3 and generally a small amount of reverse T3 (rT3). Reverse T3 has no biological activity, but it's essential to slow down metabolism as a natural compensatory mechanism during starvation or famine. When you're starving, pregnant, or under a lot of emotional stress, you can convert T4 to rT3 instead of T3. Reverse T3 has a negative feedback effect on T3 and ties up thyroid receptors, having a net effect on your body of low T3 no matter what your actual levels are.

If your lab results show a profile of low or normal free T3 levels; elevated rT3; low, normal, or even increased (although rare) T4 levels; and normal TSH, you will most likely benefit from thyroid replacement. The type of thyroid medication you take is important, however, because rT3 must be displaced by biologically active T3, not more T4 (which can convert to more rT3), if metabolism is to be normalized. Refer to the section "How to Fix It: Your Thyroid Hormone Treatment Options," later in this chapter, for more information. This low T3 syndrome occurs in numerous acute and chronic diseases not directly related to actual pathology of your thyroid gland.[15]

Thyroid Hormone Resistance

Lastly, a condition that has been getting a lot more attention recently is something called thyroid hormone resistance. In this condition, some or all of the tissues of your body and brain are resistant to thyroid hormone and don't respond normally to it. Because of this, your metabolic rate is not sufficient even though your hormone levels are normal (or even on the high side) when tested.[16] The solution to this problem is also to supplement thyroid hormones to overcome the resistance. Looking at symptoms is the only way thyroid resistance can be detected. It's thought that a large percentage of fibromyalgia cases are due to this condition.[17]

My Test Results

I had a lot of the deficiencies and conditions listed in this section, including very high levels of mercury and cadmium. The high levels of mercury may have stemmed from environmental exposure. I lived in the Philippines for six years in junior high school and high school, where my father served as a diplomat. I had to get four shots every six months (typhoid, typhus, etc.) that contained a mercury preservative commonly used in vaccinations and other medicines. I also drank the city water, which had no environmental controls, such as heavy metal or chemical dumping restrictions. Since all of my four siblings also have fairly serious endocrine deficiencies, it is likely that we had some detrimental environmental exposure coupled with a genetic predisposition for neuroendocrine problems.

My diet had also resulted in many vitamin and mineral deficiencies. I had become a vegetarian by the time I was in my late 30s because I had a hard time digesting meat, but I hadn't figured out how to get proper protein on a vegetarian diet and ate mainly pasta. Stress was a fact of life with my career, and my liver function was very sluggish (as good thyroid function is necessary for the liver to work well).

My tests showed low normal levels of TSH and T4, yet virtually no T3, clearly demonstrating a lessened ability of this conversion mechanism, as well as problems with my hypothalamus or pituitary. So, how do we increase the conversion of T4 to T3? Get levels of vitamins, minerals, and heavy metals tested, supplement vitamin and mineral deficiencies, and work with your doctor to rid yourself of excessive heavy metals. Don't "diet." Eat a balanced diet of fats, carbs, and protein. Cut out, or cut down on, alcohol. Get regular exercise, if possible, to reduce stress. It's important to note that your problem may be too long-standing to reverse itself completely (mine was) when you correct deficiencies and remove any toxic burden. But don't get discouraged—supplementing with the right kind of thyroid hormones will resolve the deficiency of T3.

Tyler, Kyle, and Myles' Story

I have unfortunately passed along my genetic heritage to my sons. This is something we must be on the alert for, as it's much easier to intervene and change the course of history when our children are young than after many years of thyroid malfunction. I have three boys, currently aged 20, 15, and 13. They all have thyroid dysfunction, although, interestingly, each has a very different problem.

Tyler

My oldest son, Tyler, has always had symptoms similar to mine—chronic sinusitis and bouts of constipation—since he was very young. At age 17, he also started to have problems with concentration and memory, and his friends kidded him that he had ADD. Given my family history, I was aware that there was a good chance my kids might have thyroid problems. When Tyler went to college and was having a hard time concentrating, I started him on a trial course of Armour thyroid, but it made him tired and didn't help with the cognitive issues. I didn't have a chance to measure his levels since he was out of town, so I wasn't sure what was going on.

When he came home for the summer, he confessed that he was feeling worse (more brain fog and confusion) and worried about keeping up in school next fall. His congestion had gotten so bad that he had a hard time breathing well when lying down, and it was interfering with his sleep. I tried Armour thyroid one more time, with no better results.

We did a battery of tests on him and found several things: His endocrine system was not very robust. Many of his hormone levels were low, including testosterone and growth hormone, suggesting that he wasn't getting enough stimulation from either his thyroid, pituitary, or hypothalamus. His thyroid levels all looked good; his TSH wasn't too high or too low and his free T3 and T4 levels were fine.

One thing was way out of line, though. His reverse T3 was very elevated. Read "What Is Reverse T3?" in this chapter, and you'll learn that reverse T3 (rT3) effectively blocks the action of T3 and renders it useless. This explained Tyler's symptoms of profoundly low thyroid even though his T3 levels were in the middle of the testing range.

When a thyroid product has T4 in it, it can simply convert to more rT3, compounding the problem. If your rT3 level isn't too high, a combination T3/T4 drug may work fine. But for my son, the problem was so severe that he couldn't tolerate any additional T4. The solution to this problem is to supplement only T3.

Tyler started on 5 mcg (micrograms) of Cytomel, a T3-only thyroid drug, and his response was immediate. His mind was completely clear from the first day, and he was noticeably more cheerful and optimistic. His sinus congestion cleared up after about a week and has been absent ever since. He has not had this long a period without sinus problems in more than 10 years. His skin has also cleared up after many years of sunspots and dry skin.

Kyle

My second son, Kyle, who's 15 years old, has an even stranger thyroid history. Two years ago he started to develop symptoms of hyperthyroidism. His right eye started to bug out (called exophthalmos), he was very nervous and agitated, he couldn't sleep, his hands trembled, and he had diarrhea and sweated constantly. I took him to a pediatric endocrinologist who ran tests that showed that he had elevated thyroid stimulating hormone receptor (TSHr) antibodies, and he was diagnosed with Graves' disease. The doctor then said my son's treatment options were either to drink radioactive iodine or take drugs to slow down his thyroid.

The problem I saw with these two options was that while the concept of radioactive iodine may sound effective—it's supposed to be actively attracted to the thyroid gland, which it seeks out and slows or kills—when you apply common sense to this equation, you realize that the radioactive material does not stay confined to the thyroid (as evidenced by the fact that after drinking it, patients must be quarantined for several days because they are actually radioactive and can harm all around them). The drug approach to slow down thyroid function also has many side effects, such as liver damage, anemia, joint pain and swelling, and inflammation of the blood vessels, so it was a scary option—it could have affected Kyle's health for the rest of his life.

Faced with these two options, I immediately turned to my endocrinology research books. I have found that the endocrinologists from the 1800s and early 1900s were remarkably rational in finding solutions that supported their patients' entire endocrine system, resulting in overall health. They didn't have pharmaceutical products to fall back on to treat symptoms, so they had to try to cure their patients' diseases.

What I found was exciting. In 1903, Charles Sajous, M.D. wrote in Internal Secretions and Principles of Medicine that Graves' disease was caused by an oversensitivity of the central nervous system (CNS), usually genetic. This oversensitivity was then aggravated by toxins of some sort that were generally of an intestinal nature or triggered by strep or some other infection. His belief was that this CNS aggravation results in overstimulation of endocrine organs (such as adrenal, thymus, or thyroid) and excessive hormone production.[18]

Kyle had mononucleosis just prior to developing his hyperthyroid symptoms, and he also had chronic ear infections when he was young. He was treated with antibiotics constantly for many years, topped off with two sets of ear tube surgeries to facilitate drainage. I look back now and realize that his intestinal balance was probably compromised, as he craved sugar while very young, probably caused by the chronic antibiotic treatment, which caused gut dysbiosis, or imbalance of the intestinal flora. But whether it was this or the mono, or something else, the treatment is the same.

Dr. Sajous goes on to say that the best way to treat this overstimulation is with thyroid therapy. He said that the disease has three *distinct phases, and that you have to be very cautious using thyroid therapy during the very early stage as it would be like "adding fuel to the fire." But in the second stage, which involves obvious excessive thyroid activity and symptoms, thyroid supplementation had proven effective in calming thyroid activity.*

I figured as this had been tried and found successful a hundred years ago by a large number of people, it was certainly worth a try before moving to the other two, more unpleasant, options. Fortunately, I have made hormone converts out of many doctor friends along my path; one of them listened to my research, found it believable, and prescribed Armour thyroid.

The result was everything I had hoped for. It was almost impossible to believe, but his symptoms resolved in two days except for the exophthalmos condition of his eye, which took a couple of months to resolve. He has been using this treatment for almost two years and it continues to control all his symptoms. Subsequent lab tests haven't revealed antibodies, so this treatment seems to have calmed down the autoimmune activity. We have tried to stop the treatment several times, and his symptoms come right back. I am hoping that after he gets through puberty and his hormones settle down, the condition might resolve itself, but I am grateful he has not had to resort to the other, more toxic, treatments.[19]

Obvious to say, but this path is fraught with risk and must be monitored closely by a doctor. As I mentioned previously, it could exacerbate a hyperthyroid condition just as easily as it could resolve it.

Myles

My 13-year-old son's story is not quite as dramatic, but profound nonetheless. He started to struggle academically in second grade. His teacher told us that he should be evaluated for learning disabilities, as he was smart but was having a hard time understanding instructions, and that he might have some sort of learning disorder that required special attention. He had wet his bed at night much longer than normal and he was also very emotional and burst into tears at the least provocation (both signs of hypothyroidism).

He responded beautifully to low-dose Armour thyroid treatment. His teacher couldn't believe the turnaround. He's been at the top of his class ever since, and the tears and bed-wetting stopped almost immediately.

That's the saga of the Simpson children. I won't go into my husband's story, but needless to say, it took two of us to create such a complex thyroid heritage. He's also on Armour thyroid, and at 55 has already avoided his father's fate of a fatal heart attack at 51. Now that we know that heart health depends on thyroid health, we are planning on his living to a healthy old age. Taking testosterone and thyroid replacement, he feels great and plays tennis aggressively three times a week without the aches and pains that used to slow him down. (And he now actually wins sometimes!)

The Role of Thyroid in MS: Study Findings

Thyroid hormone is essential for normal nervous system functioning. Studies show that thyroid dysfunction is much more common in people with multiple sclerosis. These abnormalities include hyper- and hypothyroidism, as well as antithyroid antibodies (mainly thyroglobulin and microsomal).[20] The main finding, however, was that *T3 levels were significantly lower in people with MS*.

- T3 levels in women and men with MS were statistically significantly lower than in those without, but T4 levels were the same.[21] Because most doctors measure only TSH and T4, thyroid problems are often overlooked.
- Treatment with thyroid hormone during a phase of early nerve damage resulted in protecting myelin sheaths and speeding up repair of already damaged nerves, as well as helping protect against further nerve damage. Chronic disabilities in multiple sclerosis are believed to be caused by neuron damage and degeneration caused by demyelination, and studies have shown that thyroid hormone enhances and accelerates remyelination—it restores myelin sheaths and exerts a neuroprotective effect on nerves.[22]
- Thyroid hormone has a profound effect on brain development, due to its effect on remyelination. T3 is necessary in the formation of central and peripheral myelin.[23]
- Thyroid disorders are at least three times more common in women with MS than women without MS.

T3 levels in women and men with MS were statistically significantly lower than in those without, but T4 levels were the same. Because most doctors measure only TSH and T4, thyroid problems are often overlooked.

Thyroid's Relationship with Other Hormones

> *Important interrelationships exist between your thyroid and your other endocrine glands.*

Important interrelationships exist between your thyroid and your other endocrine glands. When you have hypothyroidism, this interconnection can result in one or more parts not working correctly. Thyroid function influences and is influenced by the pituitary, gonads (ovaries and testicles), adrenals, and parathyroids. The metabolic slowdown caused by hypothyroidism slows all these glands, as well, resulting in lower overall hormone production.

Your Ovaries or Testes

In earlier chapters, we discussed the relationship between your thyroid and the function of the ovaries and testes. Women's thyroids have a mutually dependent relationship with estrogen and progesterone because their ovaries have receptors for thyroid hormone, and their thyroid has receptors for estrogen and progesterone. Men have the same relationship between their thyroid, testes and testosterone. When estrogen and progesterone in women, or testosterone in men, are low, it can cause decreased thyroid function. On the other hand, when thyroid function is low, it can cause lowered ovarian and testicular activity—creating a vicious cycle. This is why it's important to test levels of all key hormones at the same time.

Your Adrenals

The interaction between your thyroid and your adrenals, and the important hormone they make, cortisol, is critical. When your body's metabolism is slowed because of low thyroid function, your adrenal function slows, too. Insufficient adrenal activity results in inadequate cortisol production, which is necessary to produce thyroid hormones and to convert T4 to T3, as well as for thyroid receptor function. The adrenal glands are discussed at length in the next chapter.

Thyroid Testing Issues

I have mentioned a bit about the complexities and drawbacks of thyroid testing. This is particularly important to understand when your lab tests are "normal" but you have many symptoms indicative of low thyroid. There are several situations that can cause this. First, the "normal" reference ranges labs use are simply guidelines; many of us require higher hormone levels to feel good. Another confounding factor is that most testing labs employ outdated reference ranges for TSH levels.[24] TSH is the primary test doctors use to evaluate thyroid function, as TSH levels rise to stimulate production of thyroid hormones as levels fall. Many of the large labs use old TSH ranges that go much higher (up to 7 in some cases) than endocrinologists currently recommend. Usually, if your TSH level is over 2.5 (or even over 2), you will probably benefit from thyroid medication, even if your T4 and T3 levels are still in "normal" ranges. Doctors who do not specialize in thyroid treatment just look at your results in relation to these ranges. If they are within the range, even if your TSH is as high as 5, they will think you have no problem and will look no further.

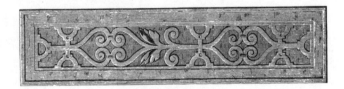

Special Situations May Require Special Doctors

If you have central hypothyroidism caused by disease or damage to your hypothalamus or pituitary, you'll need to work with a trained thyroid specialist or endocrinologist to evaluate your situation. With this condition, TSH levels are usually normal or low, T4 is reduced, and T3 is normal or reduced.[25] Even if your TSH levels are normal, the TSH molecules aren't functioning properly, which results in inadequate thyroid activity.[26] Unfortunately, most doctors who don't specialize in thyroid treatment and do not take symptoms into consideration would interpret these results to mean that you don't have a thyroid problem.

Thyroid Testing Recommendations

Your initial tests should include thyroid stimulating hormone (TSH), free T4, free T3, reverse T3, and thyroid antibodies. The *free* levels are the amount of hormone that's biologically active in your body—rather than *total* levels.

Because people with MS can have five times higher than the normal incidence of thyroid antibodies, it's important to check this out.[27] Antibody tests should include thyroid peroxidase antibodies (TPOAb), thyroglobulin antibodies (TgAb), and thyrotropin receptor antibodies (TRAb).

How to Fix It: Your Thyroid Hormone Treatment Options

Resolving thyroid deficiencies should be an integrated process. In addition to any thyroid replacement your doctor may recommend, it's always best to look at diet and nutritional aspects, as well. In order to make and utilize thyroid hormones, you need adequate levels of iodine, tyrosine, selenium, B complex (B6 is critical), zinc, manganese, magnesium, and chromium.

You should be conscientious about your diet, as well. This does not mean restricting anything that looks or sounds good; it simply means choosing good-quality sources of protein, fats, and carbohydrates (complex, *not* simple—as in brown rice, not white). It also means restricting alcohol as much as possible.

Resolving thyroid deficiencies should be an integrated process. In addition to any thyroid replacement your doctor may recommend, it's always best to look at diet and nutritional aspects, as well.

Once you and your doctor have determined the need to try thyroid hormone, selecting the right kind of thyroid medication is extremely important.

The Most Commonly Used Thyroid Medication

The medication most commonly prescribed for hypothyroidism is synthetic T4 thyroid hormone, or levothyroxine (brand name Synthroid). With a huge marketing budget behind it, Synthroid has been the second-highest-selling drug for decades in the U.S.

This drug may be effective for some, but in my experience with those who have MS, a mixture of both T3 and T4 is often a better option. The deciding factor should be your individual levels of free T3, as well as your response to therapy. If your T3 levels are robust (they generally should be in the top quartile of the range) and you don't have elevated reverse T3, your doctor may want you to try T4 therapy first. If this doesn't completely resolve your symptoms, it's important to try a combination T3/T4 therapy to see if you get better results.

The active form of thyroid hormone, T3, is required for use in our cells and tissues. In order to obtain T3, when we use a T4 medication, we must convert the T4 to T3 in our liver and cells. Based on clinical study findings, it appears that many of us with MS can't convert the hormone very well, so if we don't use a drug with both T3 and T4 in it we may get poor results. This is also true if we are converting T4 into excess reverse T3. Adding only T4 will cause more production of reverse T3. The net result of these two situations is the same: not enough T3 to fuel our metabolic processes, control inflammation, and detoxify the body.

What I Experienced
I started out using only T4 and was disappointed with the results. I had a bit more energy and slept better, but my eyesight, bladder, pain, and other problems didn't resolve. Because my T3 level was so low, I was finally able to convince my doctor to let me try T3, too. This involved using a T3-only drug called Cytomel, along with the T4-only Synthroid.

I felt better on this combination than I had when I just used T4, but it was very hard to dose. The T3 drug is very quick acting and has a half-life of seven hours, whereas T4 has a half-life of seven days. What this means is that Cytomel raises thyroid levels very quickly, and if you use too much, it can cause symptoms of excessive thyroid, such as heart palpitations, trembling hands, insomnia, sweating, and nervousness. I went up and down over the course of the day and feel alternately that my thyroid levels were a bit too high and then a bit too low. I ended up taking multiple doses of T3 to try to keep my level stable, but this was too hard to manage. It wasn't until I started on Armour thyroid that I resolved all my symptoms. Armour is made of the entire thyroid gland (from pigs) and includes T1, T2, T3, and T4.

Glandular thyroid products made of the whole thyroid from animals have been used for more than a hundred years. Armour, the best choice of the glandular products, is dosed in grains, each of which equals 60 mg and contains 38 mcg of T4 and 9 mcg of T3.

Thoughts on Dosing

Thyroid medication dosing is completely individual. There is no way to tell what your optimal dose will be without trial and error. Test results don't help in this situation because everyone has different thyroid needs. Your optimum dose may be anywhere from 1 grain (60 mg) to 4 grains (240 mg). It is unlikely that you will need to go higher or lower than these doses; many adults take 2 grains, which is my dose. It is important to raise your dose slowly, as too much thyroid too soon after your body has been in a seriously low metabolic state for a long time can cause symptoms of *hyper*thyroidism. Most doctors recommend starting at 30 mg and raising your dose by an additional 30 mg every five to seven days. If you do get symptoms of hyperthyroidism from too high a dose, you will have to decrease your dose until they subside.

> *Thyroid medication dosing is completely individual. There is no way to tell what your optimal dose will be without trial and error.*

You will most likely feel some benefit from a particular dose for a couple of days (unless it is way too low) and then slowly start to lose the benefits. This is to be expected as your body's metabolism has moved up a notch—and when it's adjusted, it wants more. This process of slowly inching up your dose continues until you start to feel the loss of benefits, or maybe even have signs of too much hormone, such as heart palpitations and trembling hands. These symptoms can mean either that you have hit your limit or that your body, having been hypometabolic for a long time, needs to adjust to a higher level of stimulation. You will need to work closely with your doctor to titrate to your optimal dose but I found in my personal situation that these symptoms generally subsided quickly. When I finally got to a dose when they didn't subside after a couple of days, I lowered my dose by 15 mg. and I was fine from then on. It's obviously important to keep your doctor apprised of all changes during this titration process.

A Few Pointers

When you are as low in thyroid hormone as I was, you are very sensitive to changes in levels that result from inconsistent potency in the product. What I found was that it's important to be sure you are getting consistent effects from one month's prescription to the next. This might sound intimidating, but it's simple once you get the system set up.

I use only "brand" Armour thyroid. Because it's one of the cheapest drugs around, it shouldn't pose a financial hardship for anyone. In fact, always ask the pharmacy what your cash price is, as it's often cheaper than insurance co-pays—less than $20 for a month's supply.

I learned the hard way that most pharmacies buy large containers of Armour thyroid (1,000 tabs) and then dispense out of this container. The problem is that when this container is continually opened and exposed to humidity and light, the thyroid hormone can degrade. The solution is easy. I ask my pharmacist to order a sealed 100-tab bottle from Forest Labs (the maker of Armour thyroid), which is the smallest container the company makes. This way it's always fresh, with good potency. Storage and transport is also important. You should store it where it doesn't get too hot or too cold; when you fly, don't check it with your bags, as the temperature in the baggage compartment can affect it.

Many doctors believe you should take your thyroid medication as soon as you wake up in the morning, at least a half hour before you eat, and that it is better assimilated if you chew it. It has a sort of sweetish taste, which isn't bad, so try it. You shouldn't take calcium or iron supplements or antacids within two hours of taking thyroid medication, as they interfere with its effect (this means no orange juice with added calcium, as well).

When you start thyroid therapy, you need to be on the lookout for low adrenal function. It has the potential to compromise your thyroid therapy.

And finally, here's an issue that's so important that it appears several times in this book: When you start thyroid therapy, you need to be on the lookout for low adrenal function. It has the potential to compromise your thyroid therapy. When you supplement thyroid hormones, your metabolism starts to speed up, and if you have poor adrenal function (read the next chapter to fully understand this concept), it may prevent the thyroid therapy from working. I experienced this phenomenon, and it can be very confusing if you're not watching for it. Several things can signal that your adrenals need help:

- The thyroid replacement may either not seem to work at all from the start, or you may have symptoms of thyroid overdosage on very low levels of replacement. If either circumstance occurs, you will need to stick to it and continue your detective work (as annoying as this prospect sounds, it's worth it). Your adrenal function will need to be evaluated, and if low, supplemented with a glandular adrenal product or bio-identical cortisol; otherwise, you won't be able to benefit from the thyroid therapy. Checking cortisol levels before you start is important, as it will give you an indication as to whether you have an adrenal problem. If your cortisol levels are low, you should talk to your doctor about cortisol replacement (see Chapter 6) when you start thyroid medication.

- If initial cortisol levels are not drastically low, it doesn't rule out your needing adrenal support. Here's why: When your thyroid function is very low, your adrenal glands don't receive enough metabolic support to work properly. Without enough thyroid stimulation, your liver is also unable to work properly. Your sluggish liver can't clear cortisol from your body effectively, leaving you with artificially elevated levels of cortisol on tests. When your liver speeds up under the influence of thyroid, it clears cortisol quickly from your body and your adrenals, which are used to working in slow motion now can't make enough cortisol to replace levels fast enough, leaving you with a shortfall.

- You might feel good for a week to several weeks and then get to a thyroid dose that increases your metabolism significantly. All of a sudden, your symptoms start to come back. You try raising your thyroid dose and you feel worse. This scenario signals that your adrenals aren't up to the new, increased demands of your body, which is finally working as it should. At this point you *must* address this adrenal deficiency in order to be successful with your thyroid therapy.

Key Points

- Your thyroid regulates transport of raw materials (such as glucose, oxygen, and enzymes) into your cells to produce energy. Just as important, it regulates transport of the waste products from this energy production process back out. These two processes of energy production and detoxification are critical to health.
- Most of the symptoms of MS are well-known symptoms of hypothyroidism. To get to the bottom of what's going on in your personal situation, you must evaluate your symptoms as well as measure levels of thyroid hormone using lab tests.
- Many different things can go wrong with your thyroid, leading to the symptoms of MS. It's important to evaluate your thyroid as thoroughly as possible to determine whether thyroid malfunction is the cause of any of your symptoms.
- Clinical studies have proven that the thyroid is essential in nerve health and repair, and that it has the potential to restore myelin damaged in MS.
- To get an accurate understanding of your thyroid function, you must test free T3, free T4, TSH, reverse T3, and thyroid antibodies.
- It's important to use a T3 hormone product (preferably Armour) if you have low T3 levels and/or high reverse T3 levels (which may require a product with only T3).
- Do not start on thyroid hormone therapy without first evaluating your adrenal function by measuring cortisol.

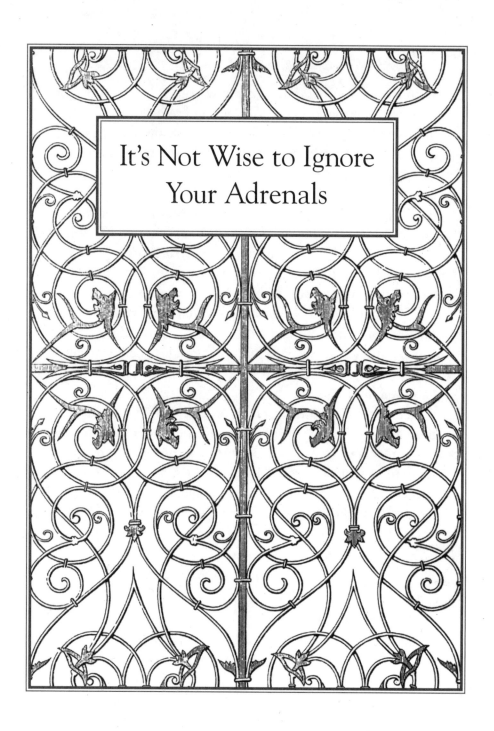

VI

What Do Your Adrenals Do?

You have two adrenal glands, each situated directly above a kidney. These tiny glands make several critical hormones, including cortisol, adrenaline, and DHEA (dehydroepiandrosterone). Cortisol helps regulate your immune response, assists your body in using sugar and protein for energy, and helps you recover from infection and stress, which is why it's known as a stress hormone. In other words, it's produced when you are under stress, either physical or emotional.

In response to a stressor, our bodies go through profound biochemical changes. First, you make greatly increased amounts of cortisol. Second, functions that aren't essential to survival are curtailed, such as blood flow to nonessential areas, including hands, feet, scalp, and intestines; this disruption in blood flow causes digestion to slow so that your body can redirect its resources to deal with the emergency. This reaction results in an increase in heart and breathing rates, blood pressure, body temperature, and levels of fat and sugar in the bloodstream. It quickens the brain and increases muscle strength and energy—all necessary to survive a crisis.

Cortisol is critical in controlling the chronic inflammation found in MS, yet clinical studies have shown that people with MS are less sensitive to the cortisol they produce.

Unfortunately, the other, less critical challenges of daily life are also enough to provoke increased cortisol production. Just the frustration of dealing with the physical challenges of MS, not to mention having to fight continuous inflammatory activity, is enough to wear your adrenals out. If excess cortisol production continues, it can damage your immune system as well as cause other negative health impacts, including increased blood pressure, cholesterol, triglycerides, and blood sugar levels.

Your Adrenals and Multiple Sclerosis

The ongoing physical and mental challenges we experience when we have MS cause chronic stress. When you experience an exacerbation, a transient period of severe symptoms, your body produces enormous amounts of cortisol to try to resolve it. This is why doctors prescribe extremely high doses of synthetic glucocorticoids (a non-bio-identical version of cortisol) when we're having a relapse. It reduces inflammatory activity immediately. The downside is that high-dose steroid therapy like Solu-Medrol has many negative side effects, such as cataract formation, gastrointestinal bleeding, osteoporosis, and diabetes, so it's not a good long-term solution to controlling inflammation.

After an extended period of excessive cortisol production, your adrenal glands become fatigued and can't make enough cortisol any longer. Because cortisol suppresses autoimmune reactions and inflammation, decreased cortisol production compromises your immune function and can result in increased autoimmune activity and disease progression. Cortisol is critical in controlling the chronic inflammation found in MS, yet clinical studies have shown that people with MS are less sensitive to the cortisol they produce.[1] In postmortems, adrenal glands of people who had MS were found to be enlarged, demonstrating there was a period of excessive activity at some time, possibly resulting in their losing sensitivity to cortisol.[2]

This situation is not fully understood yet, but we do know that prolonged high cortisol levels can affect the feedback loop with the hypothalamus and pituitary. These glands regulate your adrenals just as they do your other endocrine glands. If cortisol is too low, they release hormones to increase levels, and if it's too high, they tell the adrenals to slow production. If something goes wrong with the feedback loop (as with the thyroid in central hypothyroidism), cortisol levels, as well as the cortisol receptors present in almost every cell in your body, are affected; then you can't make or utilize enough cortisol to keep inflammation and autoimmune activity in check.

In many with MS, this feedback system doesn't appear to work properly. These findings suggest that increased hypothalamus, pituitary, and adrenal activity is followed by a reduction in cortisol sensitivity, and when this mechanism doesn't work, it affects your body's ability to control inflammation.[3]

An interesting finding is that when optic neuritis, a fairly common symptom of MS, is treated with cortisol as soon as

There is certainly enough proof of adrenal involvement in MS to suggest that everyone diagnosed with MS, or anyone who exhibits MS symptoms, should have their cortisol levels tested.

it's detected, the chance of developing MS decreases, showing the importance of cortisol in the MS disease process.[4] There is certainly enough proof of adrenal involvement in MS to suggest that everyone diagnosed with MS, or anyone who exhibits MS symptoms, should have their cortisol levels tested.

How You Produce Cortisol

Not only is the amount of cortisol you're making important, *when* you make it is just as important. Every hormone has its own distinct production pattern. Most hormone levels are higher in the morning and lower at night (except for one or two, such as growth hormone and melatonin); this pattern is called a circadian rhythm. Cortisol peaks an hour after you wake and then drops steadily all day.

Problems can occur not only when cortisol levels are too high or too low, but also when you have a disrupted production pattern. Any one of several unhealthy patterns can occur. A common one as we age is to have too low levels during the day and then excessive levels at night. This fluctuation results in having a hard time getting started in the morning and then feeling better as the day progresses. Cortisol is the only hormone that actually increases as we age, and at night, cortisol levels are an average of 10 to 12 times higher for a 50-year-old than for a 30-year-old.[5] Increased cortisol doesn't lend itself to a good night's sleep. This demonstrates why it's important to measure your cortisol levels several times during the day to get an accurate picture of your production pattern.

> *It's important to measure your cortisol levels several times during the day to get an accurate picture of your production pattern.*

Healthy Daily Cortisol Production Pattern

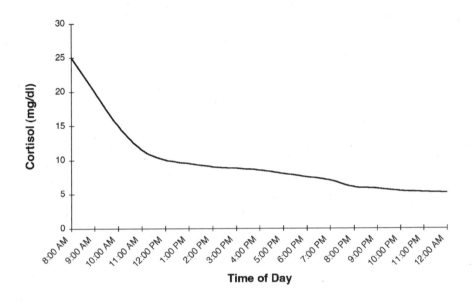

What Can Go Wrong With Your Adrenals?

Loss of adrenal function, which many of us with MS experience, can be a long, drawn-out process or a quick, brutal one. A very traumatic event or illness can deplete your adrenals rapidly. On the other hand, it might take a long time for your adrenal function to become compromised.

Illness or stress causes your adrenals to mobilize cortisol to help you cope. When the stress or illness ends, your adrenals settle down. If more stress continues to bombard you, over time your adrenals actually enlarge to increase their hormone output. Depending on how healthy your adrenals (and your other endocrine glands) are, you can keep this up for years. But

As well as excessive stress, dropping estrogen levels in women or testosterone levels in men can initially cause elevated amounts of cortisol and result in symptoms such as anxiety, insomnia, and weight gain. When you go to your doctor for these symptoms, he or she will generally prescribe antidepressants. These drugs may help with the symptoms but won't fix the problem.

even the healthiest among us will finally wear down and our adrenals will get tired. The final blow that sends your adrenals into exhaustion can be a major trauma like a car accident or divorce, but usually it's less dramatic, such as a chronic condition like MS, hypothyroidism, or even a long-term dental infection.

What Happens When We Make Too Much Cortisol?

By the time we have MS, our adrenals are most likely pretty tired and are not producing enough cortisol. But in the early stages, you might still be making too much cortisol, rather than too little. As well as excessive stress, dropping estrogen levels in women or testosterone levels in men can initially cause elevated amounts of cortisol and result in symptoms such as anxiety, insomnia, and weight gain. When you go to your doctor for these symptoms, he or she will generally prescribe antidepressants. These drugs may help with the symptoms but won't fix the problem.

After an extended period of elevated cortisol, whatever the cause, your adrenals wear down, and this can result in adrenal fatigue. It's important to recognize the signs of too much or too little cortisol, as either can have a profound impact on your health. You can intervene and stop the process if you know what to look for.

You can do many things to combat excess cortisol and the damage it does, and even prevent adrenal burnout if you catch it in time. The primary ways are by improving diet and exercise and reducing stress. (That's easy to say, isn't it?) Simple carbs—anything with refined flour

Signs and Symptoms of Excess Cortisol

- Anxiety and irritability
- Diabetes
- Easy bruising and slow wound healing
- Elevated blood pressure
- Fluid retention
- Food cravings and increased appetite
- Gastroesophageal reflux
- Hair loss
- Hypoglycemia
- Insomnia
- Irritable bowel syndrome
- Loss of libido
- Memory and cognitive problems
- Muscle wasting and weakness
- Thin skin
- Ulcers
- Weight gain (fat buildup around the stomach)

or sugar in it—cause higher insulin and cortisol levels. Try to cut back on these foods and alcohol as much as possible (see Chapter 8 for more information on this). Also try to eat more frequent, smaller meals, and exercise regularly. For the solution to dropping estrogen and testosterone levels, see chapters 3 and 4 for hormone replacement options.

What Happens When We Make Too Little Cortisol?

Some of the symptoms of adrenal fatigue and low cortisol production are the same as those of hypothyroidism. The two conditions are so closely intertwined that it's often difficult to tell which is causing your problems. The answer is often that it's both, as low cortisol production is common in hypothyroidism and normal production often returns after thyroid supplementation. If the adrenal fatigue has been going on for too long, you may have to supplement with low-dose cortisol, which can restore your immune function and slow down or halt autoimmune activity.

Signs and Symptoms of Adrenal Fatigue

Which of these symptoms looks familiar? Put a check mark next to any you've experienced.

- __ Accelerated aging
- __ Allergies and/or asthma
- __ Avoidance of exercise
- __ Bowel problems including diarrhea
- __ Cheeks or eyes appearing sunken
- __ Chronic fatigue
- __ Chronic or severe sickness or infections
- __ Cold, clammy sweats
- __ Cold extremities (hands and feet)
- __ Dark circles under eyes
- __ Depression and/or anxiety
- __ Diagnosed with an autoimmune disease
- __ Difficulty processing information
- __ Dry, thin skin
- __ Eczema or psoriasis
- __ Environmental sensitivities
- __ Excessive drinking or alcoholism
- __ Eyes have become sensitive to light
- __ Feeling of shivering or shaking inside
- __ Food cravings for salt or sugar and/or hypoglycemia
- __ Groin pain
- __ Headaches
- __ Heart palpitations
- __ Inability to deal with stress (feeling ill or shaken after a stressful event)
- __ Insomnia
- __ Irritable bowel syndrome
- __ Low blood pressure and/or weak or slow pulse
- __ Low libido
- __ Memory problems
- __ Muscle and joint pain and weakness
- __ Neck and back pain and stiffness
- __ Noises in ears
- __ Pale face and lips
- __ Panic attacks and/or anxiety
- __ Temperature intolerance (cold or heat)
- __ Thinning and loss of body hair
- __ Unexplained weight loss
- __ Upset stomach and/or abdominal pain

What's DHEA Got to Do With It?

Both men and women also make a hormone called DHEA in their adrenal glands. Like all hormones except for cortisol, DHEA production starts to decline in your late 20s. DHEA has many important functions very similar to cortisol. Evidence shows that it affects your immune function and helps you withstand viral and bacterial diseases.[6] DHEA replacement has shown promise in treating lupus and HIV infection. People with chronic inflammatory disease have lower levels of DHEA. It has proven to have potent anti-inflammatory properties and has successfully prevented the development of the animal model of MS in many studies.[7]

A number of things lower DHEA levels. First and foremost is stress, either physical or emotional. When your adrenals focus their activity on producing cortisol to deal with excessive stress, DHEA production drops off.

People with chronic inflammatory disease have lower levels of DHEA. It has proven to have potent anti-inflammatory properties and has successfully prevented the development of the animal model of MS in many studies.

The Relationship Between Cortisol and Thyroid Function

When you supplement thyroid hormone and you reach your optimum dose, your metabolism will speed up. This often results in cortisol falling too low. With increased thyroid stimulation, the liver starts to function properly and clears cortisol from your body more quickly. Your tired adrenals can't make enough to keep up with day-to-day requirements, let alone make enough reserves for the challenges of MS.

Betsy's Story

Betsy was 29 when she was diagnosed with MS. It came as a shock, as no one in her family had ever had a neurological disease and until two years earlier she had been very healthy. Her symptoms started about nine months after she had her son at age 27. The overwhelming fatigue didn't concern her at first—after all, she had a newborn, didn't she? As each day dragged by, she thought she would certainly regain her strength. Her ob-gyn was very encouraging, telling her not to worry, as this was extremely common.

Over the next six months, Betsy started to notice other worrisome symptoms. The most troubling was shooting pain in her jaw. She'd sometimes get a stabbing, electric-shock-like pain on one side of her face when she brushed her teeth or put on makeup. It was always unexpected, and she was never sure what caused it. She put up with it for a couple of months, and then, figuring it must be a problem with a tooth, she went to her dentist. Her dentist took X-rays and examined her teeth and told her he had no idea what was causing it, but that he was positive it wasn't a problem with her teeth.

The next two symptoms came at the same time and convinced Betsy she had to get serious about what was going on. First, she woke up one morning and found that she had blurry, double vision in her left eye. In the next few days as she was trying to decide what to do about her eye, she started to get muscle spasms in her left leg several times a night. Not knowing what else to do, as she had never gone to a doctor other than her ob-gyn, she called him for suggestions. After hearing of her symptoms, he reassured her that she probably just had a virus of some sort, but he also referred her to a neurologist for an evaluation.

The neurologist examined her and scheduled her for MRIs of the head, neck, and spine, a spinal tap, and evoked potential tests. When Betsy went back to discuss the results, the neurologist sat her down and told her that unfortunately everything looked conclusive for MS. Starting with the pain in her face, which he told her was something called trigeminal neuralgia (a condition not uncommon in MS), all her symptoms were those of MS. He said that she was in the very early stages of the disease, but that she needed to take her condition seriously. He recommended that she have a full physical because she hadn't had one since she was a teenager, and that she do everything she could to take care of her overall health, as there was nothing that could really be done for the MS other than the "ABC" drugs (Avonex, Betaseron, and Copaxone), which he encouraged her to consider taking. All these drugs involved injections, and Betsy was deathly afraid of needles, so she decided to schedule an appointment for a full physical first.

Betsy got lucky when a friend referred her to a very forward-thinking doctor. He started the appointment by asking her an enormous number of questions about her health history, beginning with her age when she started her menstrual cycle and ending with a full evaluation of her family's health history. After they were finished, he told her that he saw some interesting trends.

First, both her mother and aunt had several miscarriages and went into menopause very early. Betsy had two miscarriages before her son was born, and she had to use supplemental progesterone to support the pregnancy to full term. She also had to use fertility drugs, as she had a hard time conceiving. He said in his experience, fertility problems as well as miscarriages could very well indicate a thyroid problem, and that fatigue was also often related to low thyroid function. When he tested Betsy's thyroid, she had normal levels of TSH but very low T3 and T4 levels, indicating a problem with her pituitary. She also had unusually low levels of estrogen and progesterone, indicating deficient ovarian function, like her mother and aunt.

He started her on Armour thyroid, a combination T3/T4 drug, and a low dose of estrogen, with progesterone to be added the last two weeks of her menstrual cycle. Her fatigue got much better immediately. She also noticed that her vision was a bit better and the muscle spasms were far less frequent. As she slowly raised her dose of Armour Thyroid, she got better and better.

After about a month, though, Betsy started getting tired in the afternoons again and her vision worsened. She immediately assumed that the drugs weren't working for her and felt completely depressed. Before she stopped the drugs, she figured she'd better let her doctor know that they didn't work for her anymore. He told her to come in right away.

He told her not to get discouraged, that what she was experiencing wasn't uncommon, and that it didn't mean that the therapy wasn't working. He said he had seen this happen in many of his patients. What was happening, he explained, was that the thyroid replacement had sped her metabolism up and her adrenals couldn't keep up with the higher demands being placed on them. He told her they needed to measure her levels of cortisol, a hormone made by the adrenals, to see if this was what was going on. He called her several days later and told her that, sure enough, her cortisol levels were very low, and prescribed low-dose cortisol for her.

She started it that day and within a couple of hours felt a difference in her energy level. Over the next week, all her symptoms began to resolve again. After several months, she still hadn't had an attack of trigeminal neuralgia and all her other symptoms had disappeared.

How to Evaluate Your Adrenal Function

Cortisol
It's important to test not only your levels of cortisol, but also the pattern in which it's produced. You can accomplish this by getting a blood test twice a day. The first test should be an hour after you get up, while fasting, and the second at about 4 p.m. to see if you are making too much or too little cortisol. Hormone expert Dr. Thierry Hertoghe says that the morning level should optimally be 18 to 20 ng/ml, and anything under 13 ng/ml should potentially be treated. And the 4 p.m. level should be 10 to 12 ng/ml, with less than 7 ng/ml being too low.[8]

Other options are a 24-hour urine test that shows how much cortisol you produce in a day (but it won't detect disrupted rhythms), or a saliva test, using samples collected four times during the day. The saliva test accurately measures your cyclic profile of cortisol by measuring levels at 8 a.m., noon, 4 p.m., and 10 p.m. This is the best option, as it shows if excesses or deficiencies exist at any of these points. See the chart in Appendix A for more information on optimal hormone levels.

DHEA
Levels of DHEA sulfate (DHEAS) should be measured. When adrenals undergo stress, levels of cortisol and DHEA are high. As they start to wear out, cortisol remains high and DHEA drops. When the adrenals finally wear out, both cortisol and DHEA levels are usually low and require supplementation.

ACTH
ACTH is a hormone produced by your pituitary that stimulates the adrenals to produce cortisol. Measuring it helps to determine if low cortisol is caused by a problem in the pituitary, which regulates the adrenals, or in the adrenals themselves. If ACTH is low, this generally

means it's the pituitary because it should have detected low levels of cortisol and increased levels of ACTH to stimulate additional production. High levels would mean that the problem lies in the adrenals, as they aren't responding to commands from the pituitary properly. This blood test should also be done as part of a thorough evaluation of your adrenal function. A further diagnostic step would be an ACTH stimulation test. In this test, cortisol levels are tested, then you're given an injection of a synthetic form of ACTH, and cortisol levels are tested 30 and 60 minutes after the ACTH is given to see how the pituitary responds.

ACTH is a hormone produced by your pituitary that stimulates the adrenals to produce cortisol. Measuring it helps to determine if low cortisol is caused by a problem in the pituitary, which regulates the adrenals, or in the adrenals themselves.

Aldosterone

Another hormone secreted by the adrenals, aldosterone, is responsible for water and salt balance in the body. When your adrenals don't make enough aldosterone, fluid is pulled out of the tissues and skin, sometimes giving your face and eyes a sunken appearance. Because aldosterone is produced by the adrenals, levels of this hormone, like cortisol and DHEA, reflect overall adrenal function. Aldosterone levels can be supplemented with a bio-identical product called Florinef if levels are too low. Measuring aldosterone requires a blood test, which should be done while you are fasting.

Treatment Options for Adrenal Fatigue

Glandular Products
Many glandular products are available at health food stores. Stay away from any that are not strictly cortisol and do not state a specific quantity. You will need to work with your doctor to find the right dose; this is a powerful substance, so your doctor must monitor it carefully, just like any other drug.

Bio-identical Cortisol
If glandular products are not strong enough and your adrenals need additional support, you should speak with your doctor about prescription bio-identical cortisol. At low doses, this treatment is often enough to support your adrenals and resolve many symptoms. Your doctor may choose to give you prednisolone or prednisone (between 2.5 and 5 mg daily), cortisol products that have been molecularly altered and have much more long-lasting effects. This may be okay for a short period of time, but it's always advisable to use the lowest-dose, bio-identical product that gives you symptom relief. The daily starting cortisol dose for women is generally between 5 and 30 mg, and for men it's 10 to 40 mg. Cortisol is taken every four hours, three to four times a day, as your body uses it quickly.

It's always advisable to use the lowest-dose, bio-identical product that gives you symptom relief.

I had to use cortisol for quite a while to rebuild my adrenal function, as my levels of cortisol were extremely low and my fatigue was overwhelming. I started at 20 mg a day on a descending dosing schedule to mimic physiologic cortisol production: 10 mg as soon as I got up, 5 mg four hours later, and 2.5 mg twice thereafter at four hour intervals.

You should feel the effects of cortisol supplementation within a few days. Adrenal deficiency is often related to thyroid deficiency, and as thyroid levels improve, adrenal function will too, usually within three or four months. You should discontinue the cortisol therapy if your levels fall within optimal ranges when measured again. You needn't worry that taking supplemental cortisol will stop your adrenal function. When you take such a low dose, your adrenals will cut back their production a little bit but they will still continue to produce cortisol. (This is also the case with thyroid supplementation.) If you have a very stressful situation (e.g., a bad flu or cold, major dental work, or surgery) while your adrenals are healing, most doctors will recommend that you increase your cortisol dose, possibly by 50 to 100%.

If you start on cortisol replacement, measure blood levels of cortisol and ACTH after 45 days and then regularly on an ongoing basis. If ACTH gets too low and/or cortisol gets too high, work with your doctor to cut back your dose. Your adrenals are one of the few endocrine glands that can heal themselves after having a chance to rest while on cortisol replacement. Therefore, try to wean off cortisol after two to three months, or if you feel that it's becoming too stimulating (indicating that your adrenal function is coming back), or if your blood levels get too high.

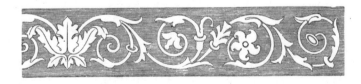

DHEA

You can buy oral DHEA over the counter, without a prescription. Men metabolize DHEA much faster than women, so they need 25 to 50 mg, while most doctors recommend 15 mg for women (unless they're being treated for rheumatoid arthritis, in which case 50 to 100 mg is recommended). Women often have difficulty with DHEA replacement, as it can block estrogen. Women with a high testosterone level must also be careful using DHEA, as it's converted to testosterone. Symptoms of DHEA excess in women include weight gain, facial hair, acne, sugar cravings, fatigue, anger, depression, deepening of the voice, insomnia, restless sleep, mood swings, and irritability. Both women and men should work closely with their doctors to monitor symptoms and blood levels.

Key Points

- Adrenal function is critical in MS and in any other autoimmune disease. The ongoing physical and mental challenges you experience with MS cause chronic stress that can result in adrenal dysfunction.
- Research shows that people with MS are less sensitive to cortisol. Also, adrenal glands are often enlarged in MS, demonstrating prior excessive activity, which is possibly what causes the adrenals to lose sensitivity to cortisol.
- Not only is the amount of cortisol you're making important—*when* you make it is just as significant. You need to test cortisol two to four times during the day to make sure that you don't have a disrupted cortisol production pattern that could be compromising your health.
- Cortisol and DHEA should be measured and replaced if low. DHEA is an over-the-counter supplement. You can use over-the-counter glandular products to replace cortisol, but you might require stronger prescription bio-identical cortisol.
- Keep a close eye on your cortisol levels and check for symptoms of low adrenal function if you start thyroid replacement therapy.

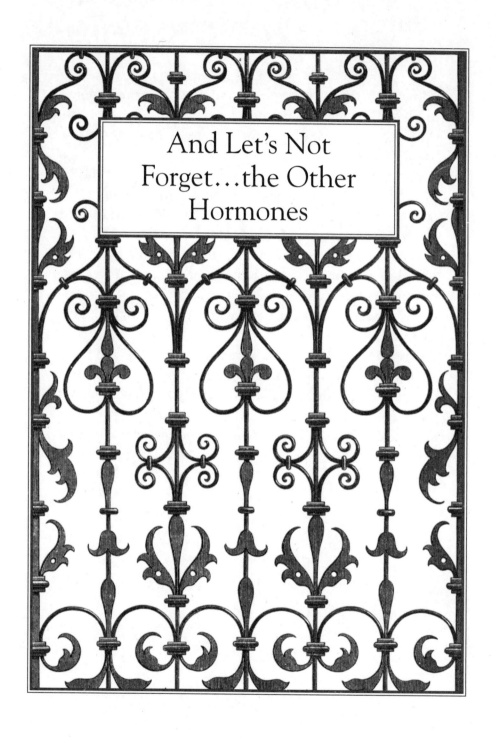
And Let's Not Forget…the Other Hormones

VII

There are several additional hormones that have been shown to have profound effects on multiple sclerosis, as they're all important in reducing inflammation and ensuring optimal immune function. These include growth hormone, prolactin, pregnenolone, vitamin D, melatonin, insulin, and parathyroid hormone. Levels of each one (except melatonin) should be measured as part of a thorough endocrine evaluation. If they are found to be deficient, they should be supplemented concurrently, as research shows that it's important to address all deficiencies in order to maintain optimal hormonal balance. Anecdotally, it has been found that lower levels of each individual hormone are needed when all deficient hormones are replaced together.

Growth Hormone—Not Just for Growth!

Growth hormone production is highest at puberty and declines progressively after age 21. Made in your pituitary, it stimulates bone and organ growth. It causes increased production and release of a substance called insulin-like growth factor 1 (IGF-1), which travels to target tissues such as bones, organs, and muscles to trigger growth and repair. It has also been shown to promote growth of myelin and nerves. Studies have found the following:

- IGF-1 promotes 20% to 30% more proliferation of the cells that make myelin, and stimulates more, and thicker, myelin.[1]
- Growth hormone therapy reduces demyelination in the animal model of MS.[2]

Growth hormone plays a big part in controlling and reducing inflammation and optimizing immune function. IGF-1 is needed to develop immune T cells and B cells, and the decrease in these important cells experienced with chronic disease and normal aging can be reversed with growth hormone replacement. Growth hormone receptors exist throughout the brain, and higher IGF-1 levels have been linked to better cognitive function, whereas growth hormone deficiency can cause poor emotional and psychosocial functioning.[3]

When testosterone in men drops, it lowers growth hormone production and results in more fat, more aromatase activity, and—you got it—more estrogen. It also decreases insulin sensitivity, which increases a condition called insulin resistance—another factor that increases fat. In this condition, your body becomes insensitive to insulin after it has been doused with too high levels for too long (usually caused by eating too many simple carbs, such as bread and pasta made from refined flour). Another dangerous effect of excess estrogen in men is an increased risk of stroke or heart attack and, the scourge of countless aging men, a swollen prostate.

Growth hormone is primarily produced in the middle of the night, so it's not practical to measure it. An accurate assessment of growth hormone status is obtained by measuring levels of IGF-1 and its binding protein, IGFBP-3. As well as being a storage protein for growth hormone, IGFBP-3 is also a hormone in its own right. It's been shown that men with lower levels of IGFBP-3 have an increased risk of prostate cancer.[4]

Many people with MS have low levels of growth hormone, and replacing levels to those of youth and health can have a profound effect on symptoms. You need to measure both IGF-1 and IGFBP-3 to get an accurate picture of your growth hormone status. The IGFBP-3 shouldn't be too high or too low. When it's too high, it binds too much of your growth hormone, which makes it unavailable for use by your body. Many doctors who replace growth hormone believe that target replacement levels of IGF-1 should be approximately 300 ng/ml.[5]

An interesting note: Research shows that in the early stages of disease, growth hormone levels go up. After a period of time, however, they get much lower than normal. Men generally lose more of their growth hormone function than women do, causing men's IGF-1 levels to be lower.[6] It's important to evaluate your endocrine function as early as possible and replace deficient hormones to forestall progressive inflammatory activity and immune dysfunction.

> Many people with MS have low levels of growth hormone, and replacing levels to those of youth and health can have a profound effect on symptoms.

Prolactin—Good or Bad?

Prolactin is a hormone made in the pituitary that plays an important role in immune system functioning. Clinical studies show that many men and women with MS have significantly higher levels of prolactin—and coincidentally, so do people with hypothyroidism.[7] People with lupus, arthritis, rheumatoid arthritis, and AIDS also often have elevated levels of prolactin.[8] It's not clear if prolactin plays a role in causing autoimmune disease or whether it's high in response to the stress the disease causes.[9]

> Clinical studies show that many men and women with MS have significantly higher levels of prolactin—and coincidentally, so do people with hypothyroidism.

There are many possible reasons for these high levels, but the first thing to remember is that all parts of your endocrine system are related and have a sophisticated system of checks and balances. If one hormone is too high or too low, it will affect many others. To give us a clue as to how to reduce prolactin, we have to investigate what might be going on in the other glands that could cause prolactin to go up.

Research shows that a drop in thyroid hormones causes the hypothalamus to stimulate prolactin. In fact, hypothyroidism is one of the main causes of high prolactin. High prolactin levels depress ovarian and testicular function and are often found in conjunction with low levels of testosterone, estrogen (in women), and progesterone. In men with multiple sclerosis, high prolactin levels are associated with high levels of estrogen and low levels of testosterone. As we know from Chapter 4, high levels of estrogen and lower levels of testosterone are major problems in men with MS. It has also been shown that pro-inflammatory stimulation of the central nervous system can increase prolactin.[10]

Treating deficiencies of these hormones may help to reduce prolactin levels and the inflammation they trigger. Levels of estrogen, progesterone, testosterone, thyroid hormones, and prolactin should be measured together. An optimal level of prolactin is 10 pg/ml.[11]

Pregnenolone—The "Mother of All Hormones"

Sometimes called the "mother of hormones," pregnenolone is the precursor, or building block, for many other hormones. Made from cholesterol, it's produced primarily in the adrenal glands, but also in smaller amounts by many other tissues and organs, including the liver, brain, skin, gonads, and even the retina of the eye.

Pregnenolone can be made into hormones such as progesterone, estrogen, testosterone, DHEA, cortisol, and aldosterone. In the past, pregnenolone was widely used to treat arthritis, as it can convert into cortisol if levels are low and reduce inflammation. Pregnenolone can also counter damage caused by excess cortisol. Cortisol is critical to health but can be toxic at higher levels. Among other things, it damages brain function, which can lead to memory problems. Blocking this process may be one of the main reasons for the well-known memory-enhancing effects of pregnenolone. You will need to monitor symptoms and levels of other hormones if you supplement pregnenolone, as women may get too high an androgen effect if it converts to DHEA or testosterone and causes symptoms such as acne, hair loss, and abdominal weight gain.

Also, studies show that pregnenolone may have a role in repairing myelin sheaths in multiple sclerosis. It dramatically improved spinal cord injuries and actually reversed paralysis when given immediately after an injury.[12] Production of pregnenolone decreases with stress, aging, depression, hypothyroidism, and toxic exposure. It can also be depleted when other hormone levels (such as cortisol) are low, as it's used to replenish supplies.

Pregnenolone levels should be tested, and if they are low, you should consider supplementing them. Pregnenolone is available without a prescription and can be found at many health food stores or online. Doses of 25 to 200 mg per day are generally considered safe, but levels should be measured after therapy starts to make sure the right dose is being taken. As with all other hormones, the lowest dose that resolves symptoms should be used.

Vitamin D—Not a Vitamin but a Vital Hormone

Vitamin D is actually a hormone, rather than a vitamin. It's made in the skin, kidneys, and liver from cholesterol with the aid of sunlight. Sun exposure alone will not make enough vitamin D. You must also be able to manufacture it in your organs, but many of us don't make enough of it to meet our needs. Many things can decrease vitamin D, including aging, use of sunblock, a low-cholesterol diet, and use of statin drugs that decrease cholesterol production. Physical or emotional stress lowers vitamin D, as cortisol is also made from cholesterol; when the body has to choose between making cortisol for survival or vitamin D, it chooses cortisol.

Research shows that vitamin D is anti-inflammatory and is good for treating all kinds of inflammatory conditions, such as cancer, autoimmune disease including MS, irritable bowel problems, and arthritis. Vitamin D receptors are present in most cells and tissues in the body, including colon, breast, lymph gland, prostate, lung, activated macrophages, and parathyroid cells. Vitamin D is one of the most potent regulators of cellular growth in cells, both normal and cancerous.[13] In a variety of animal models, it has been demonstrated that vitamin D treatment is effective in mitigating or preventing the onset of type 1 diabetes, multiple sclerosis, and rheumatoid arthritis.[14]

It has long been established that there is a geographical association with incidence of multiple sclerosis. People who were born at and lived at or below 35°N for the first 10 years of their lives have a lower lifetime risk of developing multiple sclerosis and cardiovascular disease, compared with those who were born above it.[15] When you live closer to the equator, more vitamin D synthesis takes place in your skin throughout the year, so vitamin D levels are higher.

Levels of 25-hydroxyvitamin D3 should be measured before starting vitamin D3 supplementation. Vitamin D3 has shown to be far more potent than vitamin D2 in achieving optimal replacement levels.[16] Levels should be over 55 ng/ml to ensure active effect of vitamin D in the body.[17] Most doctors recommend taking 1,000 to 4,000 IU of vitamin D3 to start. But because vitamin D is a fat-soluble vitamin, you should monitor levels while supplementing to make sure you are not

People who were born at and lived at or below 35°N for the first 10 years of their lives have a lower lifetime risk of developing multiple sclerosis and cardiovascular disease, compared with those who were born above it.

getting too high levels, which can be toxic. You may need to use Rocaltrol, a prescription drug, to give you higher levels of the active form of vitamin D if your deficiency is extreme.

Melatonin—Not Just for Sleep!

The pineal gland, located in the brain, makes the hormone melatonin. Melatonin's many important functions include regulating sleep and acting as a potent antioxidant, as well as regulating other hormonal effects. Pineal gland dysfunction and resulting low levels of melatonin have been strongly implicated in MS. Interestingly, as with many hormones, both abnormally high and abnormally low levels may cause problems.

Higher levels of melatonin may be a catalyst to triggering MS, but low levels seem to cause worse disease progression.

Melatonin production is reduced in response to light hitting the eye—with higher levels made in the dark. Some think that melatonin, not vitamin D, may be the answer to why people at higher latitudes are more prone to MS. Less sun results in too much melatonin, which in turn causes the thymus gland (which manages T cell immune activity) to allow autoimmune activity to develop. Animal studies show that constant darkness aggravates the symptoms of MS. Thus, higher levels of melatonin may be a catalyst to triggering MS, but low levels seem to cause worse disease progression. Studies show that when melatonin levels drop, it often triggers an exacerbation of MS symptoms.

One of the reasons why some scientists believe there is a link between melatonin levels and MS is that melatonin production declines rapidly just before puberty and MS starts after, possibly triggered by the drop.

A study of teenagers who developed MS at puberty showed that they had significantly lower levels of melatonin at night.[18] This drop may cause a disruption in the immune system, resulting in increased susceptibility to infection and autoimmune activity. Another study showed that MS exacerbations lowered melatonin levels, and that those with chronic progressive MS had even lower levels than those with relapsing-remitting MS.[19]

Melatonin can't be measured because it is only produced at night (unless a 24-hour urine test is done). Most of us have deficient levels after age 35 to 40 (and often even younger with MS) and can benefit from low levels of replacement. Melatonin can be purchased at most health food stores. It's important to get sublingual pills, if possible. This reduces the first-pass effect through the liver. Unfortunately, it is often sold in excessive dosages. I buy 2.5 mg sublingual pills and cut them in quarters so that I use 0.625 mg per night. Try not to exceed this dose, and try using even less first to see if you get benefit. It should also result in deeper, more restorative sleep.

Insulin—A Double-Edged Sword

Most of us don't realize that insulin is a hormone. It's released by the pancreas whenever we eat, and its job is to move blood sugar, or glucose, from the bloodstream into muscle and fat cells for storage and later use.

MS appears to have some connection to insulin abnormalities, as MS is proven to increase the risk of type 1 diabetes.

We get into problems with insulin when we eat a diet high in simple carbs: soft drinks, pasta, bread, candy, cake, pastries—you know, all the things that taste so good. These foods cause the body to produce excessive blood sugar and then more insulin to try to store it all. This eventually overloads the body's ability to manage insulin and causes the whole system to break down, resulting in something called insulin resistance. The body adopts this self-defense mechanism to survive the continual assault of blood sugar and insulin, which results in your tissues becoming resistant to insulin and leads to type 2 diabetes. Research has now proven that insulin has an inverse relationship to testosterone (in men)—in other words, when testosterone goes down, insulin goes up.[20] It is thought that insulin resistance may exacerbate cognitive problems and inflammatory responses in MS.[21] If your levels are elevated, work with your doctor to follow a diet designed to lower insulin levels (specifically, cut out simple carbs).

MS appears to have some connection to insulin abnormalities, as MS is proven to increase the risk of type 1 diabetes.[22] Research suggests that insulin is vital to normal brain functioning and that insulin problems are implicated in memory loss and neurodegenerative disorders such as Alzheimer's disease and maybe MS, so insulin levels should never be too low. Fasting insulin and glucose levels should be measured as part of a complete endocrine evaluation. Another test, called hemoglobin A1c, is also very helpful, as it gives a picture of your average blood glucose level for the past two to three months. Optimal ranges are 4 to 7 ulU/ml for insulin, 80 to 95 mg/dl for glucose, and 4.5 to 6 for hemoglobin A1c.

Parathyroid Hormone—Calcium Is Critical

Parathyroid hormone, made by the parathyroid glands attached to your thyroid, regulates the level of phosphate and calcium in your bones and blood. Low calcium causes many symptoms similar to those of MS, such as confusion and depression, as well as muscle cramping, tingling and twitching, and spasms. Your thyroid function is very important in getting the most out of your parathyroids; deficient thyroid hormone has been shown to blunt the responsiveness of bone to parathyroid hormone—clearly a danger for developing osteoporosis.

> *Low calcium causes many symptoms similar to those of MS, such as confusion and depression, as well as muscle cramping, tingling and twitching, and spasms.*

You can develop either *hypo-* or *hyper*parathyroidism. As you would expect, hypoparathyroidism results in low calcium levels, and hyperparathyroidism often causes high levels. Both are very bad for your body. Hyperparathyroidism can be either primary or secondary. In primary, which is usually caused by a growth on the glands, your parathyroids malfunction and make too much parathyroid hormone (PTH), and too much calcium results. In secondary hyperparathyroidism, low calcium caused by kidney problems or deficient vitamin D triggers your parathyroids to make excessive PTH to raise calcium levels. Often the parathyroids still aren't able to make enough and this results in ongoing low calcium levels.

Hypoparathyroidism has the opposite effect. This condition, caused by damage to the parathyroids or thyroid during surgery, an autoimmune disorder, or genetic PTH resistance, results in deficient levels of PTH and calcium. Levels of parathyroid hormone and ionic calcium (the active form of calcium) should be measured to see if either hyper- or hypoparathyroidism are causing any of your symptoms.

The treatment for secondary hyperparathyroidism caused by vitamin D deficiency is supplemental vitamin D. Hypoparathyroidism is treated with supplemental calcium, and possibly parathyroid hormone if the deficiency is severe.

Key Points

- Growth hormone plays an important role in controlling and reducing inflammation and optimizing immune function. You should have your levels of both IGF-1 and IGFBP-3 measured to determine whether you are deficient and replacement therapy might be beneficial.
- Many times prolactin levels are high in people with MS. They are often found in conjunction with low levels of thyroid hormone, testosterone, estrogen (in women), and progesterone. Treating deficiencies of these hormones can help to reduce prolactin levels and the inflammation they trigger.
- Pregnenolone is not only important in remyelinating nerves, it is also significant as a precursor hormone, or building block, for most other hormones. If levels are low, supplementing this key hormone will lead to higher levels of other hormones, as well. Measure levels before and after starting therapy to make sure your levels are optimal.

- Vitamin D is a key hormone in MS. The geographic distribution of MS has led researchers to look at vitamin D involvement in the development of the disease. It has been proven to be possibly effective in mitigating or preventing multiple sclerosis.
- Pineal gland dysfunction and resulting low levels of melatonin have been strongly implicated in MS. Available over the counter, melatonin should be used at low levels to support immune function and help normalize sleep to promote nerve regeneration and health.
- Research suggests that insulin is vital to normal brain function, and that insulin problems are implicated in memory loss and neurodegenerative disorders such as MS. Check fasting levels of glucose and insulin (as well as hemoglobin A1c) to make sure that your levels are optimum. If they are elevated, work with your doctor to change your diet to decrease them.
- Balanced levels of parathyroid hormone are essential to neurological health. If they are too high or too low, they will affect your calcium levels and can result in symptoms like those of MS. Get levels measured and supplement with vitamin D or calcium if they are low.

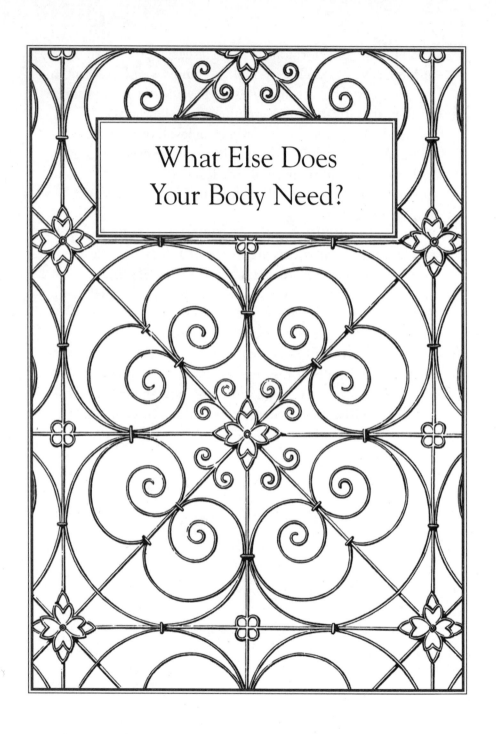
What Else Does Your Body Need?

VIII

Vitamins, Minerals, Diet, and Lifestyle: Supporting Your Hormonal Health

When we were growing up, we believed that we got all the nutrients we needed from our food; that if we ate balanced meals (with lots of milk), we were all set. This was probably more the case then than it is now, as our soil has gotten progressively more depleted of necessary vitamins and minerals due to aggressive farming practices. If you eat organic fruits and vegetables, you are in better shape to get the proper nutrients, but thousands of studies done in the last 15 to 20 years have proven that vitamin and mineral supplementation, along with proper diet, is necessary for everyone.

By the time we start to have symptoms of neurological dysfunction, we also have many vitamin and mineral deficiencies that are often caused by diet and lifestyle. Clinical studies show us that some deficiencies are common to almost all of us with MS, such as low A, B, and E vitamins; folate; essential fatty acids; magnesium; and zinc. Fixing the endocrine problems underlying our disease is our primary goal, but supporting our neurological and endocrine systems with optimal vitamin and mineral levels is also important. A good diet and the right supplements support hormone production, reestablish immune system balance, and repair and prevent further free radical damage.

What to Eat...or Not

> *Fixing the endocrine problems underlying our disease is our primary goal, but supporting our neurological and endocrine systems with optimal vitamin and mineral levels is also important.*

Every decade, it seems, there's a whole new school of thought on what to eat to stay healthy. In the 1980s, the country was swept with "fat fear." Fat would give you heart disease, high cholesterol, and even cancer and neurological disease. A common misconception was that eating high-cholesterol foods, including fats and meat, would cause cholesterol levels to go up; that somehow saturated fats would stick to your blood vessels and cause higher cholesterol levels. We gave up meat, particularly red meat; we switched to margarine; and fats, particularly saturated fats like butter, were taboo. Carbohydrates were the answer. Carbohydrates went from being a side dish, just like vegetables, to being the main course. We all started to eat lots of pasta, potatoes, bread, and salad—and most of us got sick and fat as a result. Scientific research has proven that refined carbohydrates, such as sugar and white flour, are the real culprits in increased cholesterol and disease.

All Carbohydrates Are Not Created Equal

There are two different types of carbohydrates. Simple, or refined, carbohydrates are foods made up of simple sugars in which the fiber-rich outer shell has been removed (as in brown rice to white rice) allowing them to be converted very quickly to glucose. The second type is complex carbohydrates, which are also made up of sugars, but the sugar molecules are strung together to form more complex chains. These include starches and fiber, such as whole grains, beans, vegetables, and peas. The fiber adds bulk that lowers cholesterol and also causes them to be converted more slowly to glucose, resulting in less, and slower, insulin release.

Insulin is important because the amount of insulin we make determines whether food is stored as fat or burned for energy. It's simple: The more refined carbohydrates we eat, the more insulin and glucose we produce. Our muscle cells store glucose until they get full and then refuse to accept any more. When your body releases more insulin to try to manage additional glucose, your glucose or blood sugar plunges; this is when you get the blood sugar swings that cause cravings for sugar, simple carbs, and caffeine. Because insulin problems are implicated in memory loss and neurodegenerative disorders, controlling insulin through diet is essential.

Because insulin problems are implicated in memory loss and neurodegenerative disorders, controlling insulin through diet is essential.

Refined or Simple Carbohydrates

By implementing a few basic dietary rules, you will be able to more effectively control insulin and help optimize your hormones. As hormones work together in the endocrine system, an excessive or deficient amount of insulin affects other hormones, including cortisol. The first and most important rule is to restrict refined carbohydrates severely. This means anything with white flour or sugar—you guessed it—everything we crave: sugar, cake, cookies, donuts, bread, pastry, cereals, pasta, soft drinks, even fruit juices. Always choose breads and other products that are made from whole grains instead of white flour.

It's also true that everyone digests carbohydrates at different rates, and some have much more sensitivity to them than others. I learned this unfortunate fact when I adopted a "vegetarian" diet that was 95% refined carbohydrates. I (and two of my sons) didn't gain weight, but my husband and third son gained 20 pounds each. They apparently had a greater sensitivity to the large amount of glucose that resulted from this diet, and by the time we figured out what was causing their extreme weight gain—lots of bagels and pasta—they were both on their way to becoming insulin resistant. It took almost a year to reverse the damage.

If you have sensitivity to refined carbohydrates, you are in danger of developing diabetes, a disease caused by continual strain on the pancreas because of chronic insulin production. The best way to control insulin is by restricting refined carbohydrates drastically and eating only complex carbs, such as whole grains.

Sugar
In 2003, the average consumption of sugar in the U.S. was 142 pounds per person per year, with an average consumption of 61 pounds of high-fructose corn syrup. It's in everything from soft drinks to salad dressing.[1] When we have a neurological disease, we must be vigilant about looking at labels, as sugar damages the metabolism at a cellular level and prevents the body from utilizing nutrients. It's devoid of any nutritional value, as it's been stripped of all vitamins and minerals. In order to process it, your body further robs itself of vitamins and minerals, causing further deficiencies. Low-fat foods are also often full of refined sugar, which is added to make them taste better, so people who are trying to cut back on fat are often

eating much more sugar than they realize. Excess sugar sets us up for the vicious cycle of rapidly rising and plunging blood sugar levels.

Complex Carbohydrates

Complex carbohydrates are present in fruits, vegetables, and whole grains. Because these contain more fiber, which can only partially be broken down, they result in longer-lasting energy and produce a much smaller glucose and insulin surge than simple carbohydrates do. Examples of foods high in dietary fiber include beans, oatmeal, and the skins of fruits and vegetables. High-fiber foods may be beneficial because they tend to be rich in antioxidants and low in fat and calories. A fiber-rich diet is proven to help in preventing or even reversing conditions including constipation, diverticulosis, colon and rectal cancer, heart disease, breast cancer, diabetes, and obesity.

Protein Is Important

Proteins and fats are digested even more slowly than complex carbohydrates and don't result in the same excessive glucose production. The body needs protein to get enough amino acids—the building blocks needed for almost all bodily functions, including making neurotransmitters, and the growth and repair of tissue. They provide a much slower and steadier supply of energy. Compared with the hour of energy we get from simple carbohydrates, protein provides three to four hours of consistent energy with steady blood sugar levels. With a few exceptions, animal protein is the only complete protein (which means it contains all eight essential amino acids, which are not made by our bodies

The body needs protein to get enough amino acids—the building blocks needed for almost all bodily functions, including making neurotransmitters, and the growth and repair of tissue.

and therefore must be consumed). Protein that lacks one or more essential amino acids is called an incomplete protein; most plant foods contain incomplete protein, so vegetarians need to eat a variety and balance of incomplete-protein foods (for example, combining beans and brown rice) to get all eight amino acids.

Protein is a very important element of your diet, but, as with everything else in life, it's important that you don't overdo it. Diets such as Atkins are excessive in protein and not good for us long-term. A more balanced amount of protein would be under 40% of your diet.

What Good Is Fat?

Fats have gotten a bad name in the last 20 years. The theory that the vast majority of the fat on your body comes from the fat you eat has been disproved, but it is so deeply ingrained in some of us that we have a hard time using butter or any other fat liberally. Again—too much or too little is bad for you. Americans currently get 40% to 50% of their calories from fat, somewhere in the neighborhood of 74.5 pounds per year.[2] A more balanced and healthy amount of fat would be no more than 30%.

There are two kinds of fats: saturated and unsaturated. Saturated fats include animal fats and lard, butter, coconut oil, and palm oil; unsaturated fats include polyunsaturated oils such as corn or safflower, and monounsaturated oils, including olive, nut, and canola. In moderation, all of these are critical to your body.

Fats are digested very slowly. They actually make the digestive system slow down and cause a very slow increase in blood sugar. Because of the amount of time they take to digest, they keep us from getting hungry for a much longer period of time than carbohydrates. Each gram of fat provides 9 calories of energy for the body, compared with 4 calories per gram of carbohydrates and proteins. Fats are necessary for many critical functions, including brain function and manufacturing hormones. Your ovaries and testes require a certain amount of fat in order to make estrogen, progesterone, and testosterone; in fact, cholesterol is what is used to make these sex hormones—and if you do not get enough, you may find your levels of these key hormones dropping. At a cellular level, this becomes even more important because hormones are necessary to make new cells and break down old ones. They are also necessary for facilitating your body's assimilation of fat-soluble vitamins (so, if you are taking fat-soluble vitamins such as vitamin A, D, E, or K, taking them without any fat will prevent them from being absorbed effectively).

Trans Fats

There is a class of fats—trans fats—that should be avoided at all costs. Trans fats, or hydrogenated fats, are manmade. Why would people purposefully make dangerous fats? Polyunsaturated fats are targets for oxygen, so they become rancid easily. Over 100 years ago, it seemed like a great idea to add hydrogen—in other words, to "hydrogenate" polyunsaturated fats. This prevents spoilage (a candy bar with polyunsaturated fats lasts only a few weeks, whereas one with hydrogenated fats lasts well over a year); it also makes them cheaper and easier to use for baking and converts them from liquids to solids (think Crisco). It was not realized in the early 1900s that these hydrogenated and partially hydrogenated oils raise levels of "bad" cholesterol (LDL) and lower "good" cholesterol (HDL)—a doubly damaging effect on your cholesterol. They also interfere with cellular function and block your body's use of necessary fats.

It takes a concerted effort to avoid trans fats, however, because they're everywhere. They're widely used as ingredients in processed food because they're cheaper and have a longer shelf life, and are also used instead of oil for frying in many restaurants, particularly fast-food ones, because they can

Imbalance of essential fatty acids caused by faulty lipid metabolism is common in MS and other neurodegenerative diseases. EFA deficiency causes loss of myelination, and studies have shown that fatty acids can assist in central nervous system myelination.

be used longer. For frying at home, use saturated fats such as butter (at low heat), as polyunsaturated oils can become trans fats when heated.

Essential Fatty Acids

Fatty acid imbalances and deficiencies are common in societies, like ours, that consume a lot of processed foods, simple carbohydrates, and hydrogenated fats. Essential fatty acids (EFAs) are vital for nerve and brain function because fatty acids constitute 70% of our brain and nerve tissue. They are also critical to function of the thyroid, parathyroid, and adrenals; oxygenation of cells; healthy skin and hair; metabolism and lipid regulation; hormone formation; and muscle function. In the right ratio, they are anti-inflammatory and instrumental in digestive and intestinal health and immune function.[3] Imbalance of essential fatty acids caused by faulty lipid metabolism is common in MS and other neurodegenerative diseases. EFA deficiency causes loss of myelination, and studies have shown that fatty acids can assist in central nervous system myelination.[4]

There are two EFAs that are necessary for growth and development and cannot be made by the body: the omega-6 linoleic acid, and the omega-3, alpha-linolenic acid. Our bodies make two additional omega-3 fatty acids out of alpha-linolenic acid: eicosapentaenoic acid (EPA) and docosahexaenoic acid (DHA). DHA is crucial to brain health and to the retina of the eye; ample amounts of DHA result in better cognitive and neurological function, such as memory and vision. Studies have shown DHA has beneficial effects on the heart by preventing blood clotting and high blood pressure and triglyceride levels. It has also been proven to resolve pain associated with several inflammatory conditions, including rheumatoid arthritis and inflammatory bowel disease.[5] Rich sources of omega-3s are fish oil and flaxseed oil.

The ratio between omega-3 and omega-6 is critical. Our bodies function best when our diets have a ratio of no more than 4 times as much omega-6 as omega-3, but unfortunately, most Americans eat 20 to 30 times more omega-6 oil than omega-3. This leads to increased inflammation and exacerbation of all the conditions inflammation creates—including MS. Omega-6 is found in vegetable oils such as soybean, corn, safflower, and sunflower, as well as in the processed foods made from these oils. As they're also found in the meat from grain-fed livestock, it's not hard to end up with too much omega-6, compared to omega-3.

Optimal Balance for an Optimal Diet

The right balance of fat, protein, and complex carbohydrates is critical to good health. The percent of each should be approximately:

37% complex carbohydrates (mainly vegetables)
37% protein
26% fats

The key to eating for optimal endocrine balance and support is eating all three key elements—fats, protein, and complex carbohydrates—at every meal. Eating too much or too little of any one of these things will get you into trouble. Stay away from low-fat, high-carbohydrate diets, as

An example of a perfectly balanced meal is a steak or chicken breast, brown or other whole grain rice with butter, broccoli or other non-starchy vegetables, and a salad with salad dressing containing olive oil.

they cause swings in blood sugar levels. But don't cut back completely on carbohydrates because complex carbs are an essential component of a healthy diet. They are critical to brain function, as your brain can't use proteins or fats for fuel—only carbohydrates.

An example of a perfectly balanced meal is a steak or chicken breast, brown or other whole grain rice with butter, broccoli or other non-starchy vegetables, and a salad with salad dressing containing olive oil. Try eating like this for a week and see how you feel. It should noticeably cut back on food cravings and mood swings. Once you see how good you feel, it will become easier and easier to make the right food choices.

The size of your meals and their timing are also important. Keep portions smaller and eat more often, never skip meals, and try to avoid eating a lot at night because this causes more insulin production. Your blood sugar usually gets low in the midafternoon (around 3 p.m.) and you may start to notice that you get tired and your thinking gets fuzzy. This is when you will normally reach for caffeine or sugar to give yourself an immediate lift. Unfortunately, this backfires, as your blood sugar then spikes and drops, creating a yo-yo effect.

One simple rule to follow is to eat foods as they are found in nature. If you apply this principle as often as possible, it's hard to get in trouble. And for the carbohydrates you can't seem to cut out completely, such as bread and pasta, choose whole grain instead of refined whenever you can.

Diane's Story

Diane's problems started at 38 when she went into a particularly difficult early menopause. It started simply enough with the usual hormonal challenges: She had gained an unwanted 25 pounds, started having a hard time remembering things and concentrating, lost all of her energy and enthusiasm for life, and started having chronic hot flashes and night sweats.

Within two years, it was evident that something else was going on besides just menopause. She noticed that she had begun to stumble a lot and found herself falling for no reason. At first she was sure that she had tripped on something, but eventually she realized her legs were just giving out. Next, her right hand and arm started getting numb and then it spread down her right leg, as well. When she looked down, she got a tingling feeling down her neck and the front of her thighs. When she finally went to the doctor, she was told that she needed to see a neurologist, as her symptoms were indicative of multiple sclerosis. The neurologist did evoked potential tests, an MRI, and a spinal tap, and told her there was no doubt—she had MS.

Her doctor started her on Avonex, an immune-modulating MS therapy, which gave her flu-like symptoms. These, combined with her miserable menopause symptoms, made Diane almost unable to function. She talked to her neurologist, who said she should see a doctor for the hormone symptoms, as there was no MS-related reason she shouldn't consider hormone replacement therapy.

Diane went to her GP, who ran a hormone panel. The tests showed she had very low estrogen and progesterone levels, as well as low thyroid function. She was started on estrogen, progesterone, and thyroid replacement. She hadn't really known what to expect, but it certainly wasn't a lessening of the numbness in her leg and arm. At first, she didn't really put it all together, but after a couple of weeks, there was no doubt—the numbness was almost completely gone. The therapy also had a positive effect on her energy, memory, concentration, and emotional equanimity.

Diane was so hopeful about her situation that when she started getting tired and numb again after a couple of months of hormone therapy, she scheduled another appointment with her doctor to see what was going on. Her doctor was delighted with her progress and said that there was a lot more they could do—that they had just started the process. He said he needed to ask her a couple of easy questions and then surprised her by asking what her diet was like, how much she was exercising, and how much alcohol she was drinking. When she finished answering all these questions, her doctor told her that the good news was that he thought he knew what the problem was, and there was a solution. He said that she, like so many other women her age, had a diet and lifestyle that didn't optimally support her hormones, and although hormone therapy would help, she also needed to make some diet and lifestyle changes.

Diane's diet consisted primarily of refined carbohydrates, including pasta and white rice dishes, with some vegetables and a limited amount of protein—primarily chicken. She ate virtually no fat or red meat. She skipped breakfast and had a salad for lunch, with a lot of coffee or iced tea *later in the day for energy. Her doctor said she didn't get enough protein in her diet to sustain her metabolic rate. He explained that the refined carbohydrates she was eating, such as flour and sugar, were converted quickly to glucose. Because she had too much of this sugar in her bloodstream, it was converted to fat and stored in her tissues, resulting in the weight gain over the last few years (compounded by her low thyroid function). He also told her it was extremely important to eat breakfast, because eating regularly prevents the increase in blood sugar and resultant insulin spike that occurs when you starve and then eat too much. He recommended that she cut down on refined carbohydrates and add more complex carbohydrates, such as brown rice and vegetables, plus protein and fats, into her diet at every meal.*

Next, he addressed her alcohol consumption. Diane drank two glasses of red wine four or five nights a week. She had thought that red wine was good for her heart, but her doctor explained that alcohol depletes B vitamins, which are necessary for memory and neurological function, and that women who drink alcohol regularly have been shown to have lower estrogen levels at earlier ages, bringing on menopause prematurely and making symptoms worse. He told her that it was also impossible for her to stabilize her glucose and insulin levels when she was regularly drinking wine, and that without normalized levels of these, she would never be able to optimize her hormones. He recommended that she cut out alcohol entirely if possible.

Last, he explained how important exercise is to hormone balance. Diane had told him she never had time to exercise. She couldn't fit in a trip to the gym, as she had two children still at home. Her doctor explained that one of the best kinds of exercise was something she could do right from her home—walk. It would not only help her neurologically, it would also reduce her risk of other chronic diseases, such as heart disease, high blood pressure, obesity, osteoporosis, diabetes, and certain cancers. Diane said that she could easily work this into her schedule by walking with her husband after dinner while the kids were doing their homework.

It was hard, but Diane cut out almost all refined carbohydrates and started eating a lot more meat and fats. She cut back to one glass of wine a week and went out walking in the evening when, in the past, she would have been drinking wine. It took over a month for her to detect a difference, but she started noticing that despite feeling like she was eating a huge amount because of the additional fats and protein, she got all her strength and energy back.

Some Dietary Tips

Here are some dietary suggestions everyone should consider adopting, whether they have a neurological disease or not:

- Restrict refined sugar and carbohydrates. Sugar causes vitamin and mineral deficiencies and leads to prolonged high insulin levels, which cause accelerated aging and metabolic damage.
- Eat lots of high-fiber foods. They clean out our intestines, detoxify us, and foster growth of the friendly bacteria in the digestive tract.
- Rather than the traditional three meals a day, eat four or five smaller meals containing a balanced proportion of protein, complex carbohydrates, and fats.
- Don't eat processed food marketed as "low-fat" food—they're often full of sugar.
- Eliminate artificial sweeteners. Aspartame (NutraSweet) breaks down into methyl alcohol, a poisonous chemical that has been linked to MS.
- Avoid high-fructose corn syrup, which has been proven to be more damaging to cells than regular white sugar.
- Restrict soft drinks; they leach calcium and magnesium from your bones.
- Drink eight glasses of filtered, fluoride- and chlorine-free water per day. Get a water filter for drinking and cooking. Investigate a whole-house water filter to remove chlorine from bathing water, as well.
- Reduce alcohol consumption. It stimulates insulin production and results in swings in blood sugar levels. It causes high estrogen in men and low estrogen in women.
- Don't skip breakfast. Eating regularly prevents the insulin spike that occurs when you starve and then eat too much.

- Cut back on cold drinks. The average American drinks 2 quarts of liquids a day, most of it cold. Our refrigerators are generally set at 40 degrees, which means we are drinking liquid that is almost 60 degrees colder than our body's temperature. These liquids pass around the food in your stomach and settle at the bottom of your stomach and intestines, then harden and solidify internal fat and mucous deposits—just as butter, and all other saturated fats, get hard when cold and melt when hot. This can cause the formation of stones in the kidneys, pancreas, liver, and gallbladder. Ice in beverages, by the way, is rarely used in most other parts of the world.

> *Eliminate artificial sweeteners. Aspartame (NutraSweet) breaks down into methyl alcohol, a poisonous chemical that has been linked to MS.*

- Soy products should be used in moderation. Soy is well-known to have antithyroid effects. The isoflavones in soy block the conversion of T4 to the more active form of thyroid hormone, T3. In ancient China, even though soybeans were grown extensively, they were only used as rotational crops and never eaten. It wasn't until fermentation was discovered hundreds of years later that soybeans were eaten. Other studies have determined that the phytoestrogens in soy inhibit ovarian production of estrogen and progesterone.[6] Areas of the world such as Asia that consume high quantities of soy foods have a disproportionately high incidence of hypothyroidism. People with hormone deficiencies or imbalances should avoid soy. It has the potential to disrupt ovarian and thyroid function.
- Check all breakfast cereals for the additives BHA and BHT, substances used as preservatives. The oxidative characteristics and metabolites of BHA and BHT may contribute to cancer and tumor development. There is also evidence that some people

may have difficulty metabolizing BHA and BHT, resulting in health and behavior changes. Keep these substances away from your children.
- Eat and drink organic products whenever possible, particularly meat and poultry.

Organic: Why It's Important

Many stores now label where produce is from; buy organic products from the U.S. whenever possible.

Some estimates suggest we eat approximately 15 pounds of chemicals and food additives per year, most of which comes from processed foods. They are added to lengthen the shelf life of products, make them look more appetizing, or make them taste more like the real food they are trying to mimic. Many of these substances are judged to be of questionable safety or are downright harmful.

Organic food is legally defined as food that is grown and produced without synthetic fertilizers, pesticides, use of sewer sludge (which contains substances such as cleaning products or disinfectants—whatever goes down your drain). In addition, it isn't treated with hormones or antibiotics, radiated, or genetically modified.

As our food supply gets more and more global, there are a myriad of potential problems. A large percentage of our country's produce now comes from countries that don't have the same environmental controls that the U.S. does. Mexico is a major exporter of produce to our country, and they still use DDT—outlawed in the U.S. in the 1970s because of overwhelming evidence of its toxic effects. Think about where your food comes from and what the potential health impact may be. Many stores now label where produce is from; buy organic products from the U.S. whenever possible.

Conditions Caused by Years of Low or Damaged Metabolism

After years of low thyroid function, poor diet or lifestyle, or all of the above, several opportunistic conditions can arise. They result from compromised metabolic and immune function. The most common ones follow.

Food Allergies
Many of us with MS have heard that allergies may be playing a part in our disease—most commonly to gluten or wheat. Some of the other most common food allergies are to eggs, dairy, shellfish, or foods in the potato family, which include peppers and tomatoes. These hidden food allergies can cause a large number of disparate symptoms, such as headache, sinus congestion, fatigue, stomach problems, and even depression. They can also further undermine your immune system.

It's probably wise for anyone with MS to get a complete allergy workup. Alternatively, you can try to cut out any foods that you suspect may be causing problems (or just the ones listed here that are most likely to do so). Stop eating them for 7 to 10 days, one food group at a time. If you feel worse after stopping, with such symptoms as headache, rash, or mood swings, this is an indication that they are the culprits. After this period of feeling worse, you should feel much better, and this will be your answer—you need to cut this food out and can expect a noticeable improvement in your health if you do so.

Digestion Problems
Many with long-term MS have a hard time keeping weight on even when they continue to eat the same amount. This and other things like indigestion and bowel problems are caused by the inability to digest food properly. These symptoms are caused by a decrease in production of

stomach acid and digestive enzymes. This prevents us from deriving much benefit from our food, so we become malnourished even though we may be eating quite well. You should work with your doctor to test for these deficiencies. Using betaine hydrochloride (acid) and digestive enzymes helps to increase digestion, but often this is tied to low thyroid and adrenal function, so you must test and treat these deficiencies concurrently.

Candida or Yeast Overgrowth
Candida has two forms: One is a yeastlike, sugar-fermenting organism, and the second is an infectious fungus. When our immune systems aren't functioning properly or our intestinal pH is altered, the beneficial yeast form can change to the fungal form and produce long, rootlike structures called rhizoids, which can penetrate the intestinal wall, allowing partially digested food into the bloodstream. This causes antibody formation and more autoimmune activity that further weakens the immune system. This fungal infestation can cause all kinds of illness, including "leaky gut" syndrome and irritable bowel syndrome (IBS), and allergies to food, pollen, and chemicals.

Here's an easy test to see if you may have candida overgrowth: When you wake up in the morning, before you eat or brush your teeth, work up some saliva and spit enough into a clear glass of water to cover the surface. Observe the water every 5 minutes or so for up to 30 minutes. If there are strings coming down from your saliva, if the water turned cloudy, or if your saliva sank to the bottom, you may have candida, as healthy saliva will simply float on top.

If you find that you have signs of yeast overgrowth, you should eliminate sugar and carbohydrates to starve the candida. Also, talk to your doctor about treatment options for resolving this condition. You should always have an adrenal function test if you find you have candida overgrowth, as low adrenal function is complicit in candida overgrowth.

Consistency in exercise is very important, and once you start skipping days in your routine, whether it involves going to the gym or walking around the neighborhood, you lose momentum and end up not exercising enough to provide health benefits.

It's Best Not to Ignore Exercise

Exercise is a challenge for most of us. Some of us have disabilities that prevent it, some of us are too tired, and some of us have so little free time that when we do have a minute, the last thing we want to do is spend time exercising. The solution is to find exercise that you enjoy and can realistically accomplish. For most women, a good way to do this is to combine it with an opportunity to socialize. What better way to spend an hour than in the company of a good friend walking and chatting? The trick is to find a friend who will commit to a schedule and stick to it. Men, either get out for a brisk walk or set up a gym at home that you can access easily. Consistency in exercise is very important, and once you start skipping days in your routine, whether it involves going to the gym or walking around the neighborhood, you lose momentum and end up not exercising enough to provide health benefits.

Starting with baby steps is just fine. Most of us have optimistic plans for getting in shape, which invariably involve weights, classes, trainers, etc. Then we get so exhausted thinking of all this that we end up doing nothing. Start by doing what you know you can do, and what you will most enjoy. Walking is a great activity and doesn't involve a financial commitment. Even a couple days a week is a great start.

Walking stimulates your lymph system. Swinging your arms while walking pumps lymph fluid through your system. One of the lymph system's key functions is to aid in the production of white blood cells, which destroy and remove disease-causing bacteria from your body. If you've had long-term low thyroid function, you need all the help you can get to detoxify your body.

The very far-reaching benefits of exercise are that it:

- Normalizes insulin levels
- Reduces the risk of developing colon cancer
- Shuts down the stress response, which results in lower cortisol production
- Lowers blood pressure and reduces the risk of developing high blood pressure
- Lowers blood sugar and heart rate
- Increases digestion, blood flow to the skin, and production of growth hormone
- Raises the level of "good" cholesterol and lowers the level of "bad" cholesterol
- Decreases the risk of diabetes (fit women have diabetes 66% less often than unfit women do)
- Helps build and maintain healthy bones, muscles, and joints
- Increases strength and balance (less risk of falls and fractures)
- Decreases risk of osteoporosis by promoting bone formation
- Decreases arthritis symptoms (helps keep joints flexible and helps build muscle to support the joints)

Vitamins and Minerals

I won't address the obvious minerals and vitamins we all need. It's a given that you should be taking a good multiple vitamin and mineral supplement (particularly one with all the B vitamins). Talk to the expert at your local vitamin or health food store for recommendations.

You should work with your doctor to have levels of key vitamins and minerals measured. You should do test panels for all the key vitamins such as A, Bs, C, D, and E. The following supplements are targeted specifically at neuroendocrine disorders.

Antioxidants

You should take a good antioxidant formula including the following: vitamin C, which enhances pituitary function and acts as an antioxidant (take 1,000 to 3,000 mg daily); vitamin E, which offers neurological protection (take 400 to 800 IU daily); and a good bioflavonoid supplement. Resveratrol, found in grape skins, has also been shown to be potent in reducing inflammation and boosting immunity.

Folate and Vitamin B12

Both folate and vitamin B12 are critical to nerve health, and deficiencies may cause neurologic and psychiatric disturbances, including dementia, depression, and demyelination.[7] Studies show that low B12 levels are very common in MS; they result in elevated homocysteine levels, indicating inflammatory activity and a risk factor for disease progression as well as osteoporosis and heart disease.[8] You should take folate and B12 together:

> *Studies show that low B12 levels are very common in MS; they result in elevated homocysteine levels, indicating inflammatory activity and a risk factor for disease progression as well as osteoporosis and heart disease.*

approximately 1 mg of folate and 2,000 mcg of B12. There are also skin patch B12 vitamin products available, which have been shown to work well.

Zinc

Zinc is necessary for proper immune system functioning and helps to prevent infection. Low zinc levels have been found in the central nervous system of people with MS. Zinc is a natural balance to estrogen, so it's very important for men with high estrogen levels to take because elevated estrogen has been shown to be a problem for men with MS.[9] Men with high estrogen should take up to 80 mg per day; everyone else should take 20 to 40 mg daily.

Calcium and Magnesium

Calcium and magnesium are extremely important in the development, structure, and stability of myelin.[10] Magnesium interacts with calcium and zinc, affecting the immune system and the central nervous system. It affects maintenance and function of nerve cells as well as immune system cells, so magnesium deficiency may cause dysfunction of nerve cells and the immune system. Low magnesium is thought to be a risk factor for developing MS.[11] Both calcium and magnesium have been shown to be low in the tissues of the central nervous system of people with MS, especially in the white matter area, where damage occurs.[12]

Both calcium and magnesium have been shown to be low in the tissues of the central nervous system of people with MS, especially in the white matter area, where damage occurs. Magnesium has also been shown to have a profound effect on the spasticity, numbness, and tingling commonly found in MS.

Magnesium has also been shown to have a profound effect on the spasticity, numbness, and tingling commonly found in MS.[13] A good starting dose is 500 mg of calcium and 500 mg of magnesium. When you take too much magnesium, you will experience loose bowels, so use this as a guide for your proper dose. You may need to go as high as 1,500 mg to resolve symptoms. When measuring magnesium levels, make sure that your doctor orders a red blood cell magnesium (RBC) test, as opposed to just plain magnesium. We need to make sure that levels are high enough to be getting into, and affecting, the cells. This test is the only way to measure intracellular magnesium levels.

Calcium deficiency can also cause cramping and spasticity, or tetany. Many things can lower calcium levels, including dental infections and free radicals. Ionic calcium, the physiologically active form of calcium, should be measured in conjunction with parathyroid levels because your parathyroid glands regulate calcium levels. Too high or low levels of calcium will cause neurological problems. Supplementing with calcium can resolve tetany and other symptoms of low calcium. You may have to go as high as 2,000 mg to accomplish this, depending on how low your current levels are.

Thyroid and Adrenal Support

To make and utilize thyroid hormones, you need adequate levels of tyrosine, selenium, zinc, coenzyme Q10, omega-3 fatty acids, magnesium, calcium, manganese, iodine, chromium, iron, copper, vitamin C, vitamin B (high-dose complex including B1, 2, 3, 6, and 12), vitamin A, and vitamin E.[14]

Your adrenals need vitamin C, pantothenic acid (B5), and coenzyme Q10 to function effectively.

Mitochondria Repair

Our mitochondria (the energy generators in our cells that are powered by thyroid hormone) are often damaged from many sources, a primary one being long-term hypothyroidism. It's important to resuscitate mitochondria, in conjunction with thyroid therapy, if indicated. Several substances have shown to be effective. Among them are:

- **Acetyl-L-carnitine:** Important in providing the mitochondria with fatty acids and other substances for optimum function.
- **Carnosine:** Regulates immune function so that if your immune function is low, it supports it, and if it is overactive (as in autoimmune activity), it downregulates it. It also supports your adrenal function to provide effective immune function and is anti-inflammatory and anticarcinogenic.
- **Taurine:** An important anti-excitatory amino acid. It stabilizes mitochondria and nerve cell membranes.
- **R-lipoic acid:** Repairs oxidative damage in cells and mitochondria and is critical to transport fatty acids into mitochondria. Protects the brain and peripheral nerves from damage from heavy metals and free radicals.
- **N-acetylcysteine:** Resuscitates mitochondria and protects against free radical damage.

Digestion Aids

Many of us with MS have inflammation in our GI tracts due to vitamin, mineral, and hormonal deficiencies. Using digestive enzymes, betaine hydrochloride (HCl), and probiotics can heal your intestinal lining and balance intestinal flora, resulting in better digestion and absorption of nutrients.

Key Points

- Eat a balanced diet of protein, fats, and complex carbohydrates. Try to keep the ratio of these three elements to 37% protein, 37% complex carbohydrates, and 26% fat.
- Essential fatty acids are vital for nerve and brain function. Make sure you get enough in your diet, with the right balance between omega-3 and omega-6.
- Cut back on refined carbohydrates, including sugar. Eat more complex carbohydrates with higher fiber content.
- Get some sort of exercise at least three to four times a week.
- Stay away from trans fats completely—always read ingredient lists.
- Eat organic foods whenever possible.
- Check for any underlying conditions that could be adding to the strain on your immune system, such as candida overgrowth, food allergies, or digestive problems.
- Take a good-quality vitamin and mineral supplement daily. Get levels of key vitamins and minerals measured and supplement any that are low. Adequate and balanced magnesium, calcium, and zinc are critical to symptom resolution in MS.

Final Words

A Message of Hope

I know that I've given you a lot of new information to think about and assimilate. It may seem confusing, even overwhelming at first. Don't despair. The more times you read through this book, the more sense it will start to make. It's a whole new way of looking at your disease.

First, you have to come to terms with the surprising thought that you might not be stuck with your symptoms for the rest of your life—and though exciting, it can be scary at the same time. Whenever we embark on a new therapy, all those old fears and apprehensions surface: What if it doesn't work for me? Can I take one more disappointment? Isn't it easier just to be where I am? At least I'm not in a wheelchair...or bedridden...or in a nursing home. Then there's the intimidating prospect of finding a doctor to work with: Will my current doctor be open to testing my hormone levels? Will I need to find someone new? How will I pay for it? Will my insurance cover it? Don't despair; I managed this process, and so can you.

One of the most important concepts to grasp that will enable you to stick to this path in the face of all these challenges is realizing that at the end of this process, it's possible that you will truly be *symptom free*. Once you realize that you have the potential to get rid of all your symptoms, you begin to see things in a very different light. When you replace deficient hormones and begin to feel your health returning, you realize you don't have to settle for just "feeling better" or even "okay." If, at any point, you start to feel any of your symptoms coming back—you're a bit more tired than usual, your leg gets numb again, your eyesight gets worse, or you can't sleep—you know you just have to go through a quick diagnostic check to find and resolve the problem.

By the time we get neurological problems, our endocrine systems are generally extremely depleted and our reserves are gone. We're often making very low (if any) levels of hormones so that if we don't keep our hormones at consistently healthy levels by supplementing them, our symptoms will recur quickly.

To accomplish this continuous balance, you need to set up systems to monitor and manage your hormone therapy. I keep a notebook on my desk, and every morning I write what day of my estrogen patch it is and where it's located (e.g., 0.1 mg, Day 2, on right hip; 0.1 mg, Day 3, on left hip) so that I don't get mixed up and forget to replace each patch every three days. I also note the time I take different hormones, as I tend to get busy and can forget if I have taken my progesterone, thyroid, etc.

In addition, I note which day of my cycle it is and anything I notice relative to dosing or symptoms. For instance, when I used to take cortisol, I had to take it every four hours. In the first few months of use, I noticed that sometimes I'd get tired before the four hours were up. I noted this in my notebook and after a couple of months, I realized that my cortisol wasn't high enough during the follicular phase of my menstrual cycle when I didn't supplement progesterone, and that I needed to raise my dose during this time or I would get some minor fatigue in the afternoon. I could have just accepted the fatigue, as it was inconsequential compared to what I had experienced in the past. But by this time, I realized I could feel great every day, so I analyzed my diary and realized that without supplemental progesterone I needed 5 mg more cortisol per day—and I was back to being full of energy all the time. Without writing these things down, I couldn't have figured out what was going on and resolved the problem.

Even after fours years on this path, I still have to tweak my hormone dosing from time to time. In the summer when it's warmer, I have to cut back on my thyroid dose or I get signs of excessive thyroid, such as heart palpitations; when I take progesterone two weeks out of each month, I have to ratchet back my pregnenolone dose or I have a hard time sleeping. These are minor adjustments that are individual to every person. I feel great all the time now since I realized that I never had to have a symptom again; when I do get one, I simply go through a checklist in my head and figure out what is causing it. This may seem like a pain, but when you start to feel well again, you'll realize that it's a very minor price to pay for getting your life back.

Finally, having the right advisor and advocate while you go through the start-up phase of detecting and treating your endocrine deficiencies is vital. Finding the right doctor to partner with you in this process will be critical to the success of your therapy. I will be the first to admit that this is a cutting-edge medical approach to MS; there aren't many doctors who specialize in treating hormone deficiencies, let alone have experience with using them in treating MS. You may be lucky and have an open-minded neurologist who will work with you on testing your endocrine system to see if this is a potential solution for your symptoms, but truthfully, I have found that this may not be the best medical specialty to work with on this approach. It's so far removed from a neurologist's medical training and clinical practice that it may be easier to find a forward-looking general practitioner or endocrinologist who has some exposure to hormone testing and treatment. I have included a list of country-wide doctor referral networks in Appendix B to help with this process.

You will probably need to interview more than one doctor to find the right one for you. Not only is his or her medical experience important, but it's also just as important to find someone who will be invested in working with you long-term, as *The MS Solution* can be the key to wellness for the rest of your life.

In health,
Kathryn R. Simpson

Appendix A

Recommended Hormone Serum Levels for Men

Test	Probably Deficient &/or Pathological		Optimal	Reference Range Young Adults
	Trend	Levels		
Growth Hormone				
IGF-1	Low	0-250	300-350	114-492 ng/ml
IGF-BP-3	High	>4	3	2.0-4.0 mg/l
Progesterone	Low	0-0.9	1.2	0.1-1.3 ng/ml
DHEA sulfate	Low	0-300	400	200-610 mcg/dl
Prolactin	High	≥20	10	1-19 ng/ml
LH	Low/High	≤1 or ≥6	2.0-4.0	1.2-7.4 mIU/ml
FSH	Low/High	<1 or >7	2	1-8 mIU/ml
Testosterone				
Total	Low	0-550	700	300-1000 ng/dl
Free	Low	0-180	250	50-250 pg/ml
Dihydrotestosterone	Low/High	<50 or >100	70	30-100 ng/dl
Estradiol	High	≥32	25	10-45 pg/ml
Estrone	High	≥50	40	15-65 pg/ml
SHBG	High	≥40	25-30	20-55 pmol/l
PSA				
Total	High	>5	0-1.8	<4 ng/ml
Free (% to total)	Low	0-10%	>25%	>25%

*Selected blood test data adapted with approval from *The Hormone Handbook* by Thierry Hertoghe, M.D. which can be ordered at www.imbooks.info.

Recommended Hormone Serum Levels for Women

Test	Probably Deficient &/or Pathological Trend	Probably Deficient &/or Pathological Levels	Optimal	Reference Range Young Adults
Growth Hormone				
IGF-1	Low	0-180	220-300	114-492 ng/ml
IGF-BP-3	High	>4	3	2.0-4.0 mg/l
Progesterone				
Luteal Phase	Low	0-10	13-23	3.0-27 ng/ml
Follicular Phase	Low	<1	1.4	.15-1.4 ng/ml
DHEA sulfate	Low	0-200	280	80-480 mcg/dl
Prolactin	High	>24	5.0-19	1-24 ng/ml
LH	Low/High	<1 or >12	2.0-4.0	0.2-12 mIU/ml
FSH	Low/High	<2 or >10	3.0-5.0	2-13 mIU/ml
Testosterone				
Total	Low	0-25	35	10-50 ng/dl
Free	Low	0-5	8	2-15 pg/ml
Estradiol	Low	0-120	>120	18-480 pg/ml
Estrone	High	0-60	100	40-200 pg/ml
SHBG	High	≥75	65	41-79 pmol/l

*Selected blood test data adapted with approval from *The Hormone Handbook* by Thierry Hertoghe, M.D. which can be ordered at www.imbooks.info.

Recommended Serum Levels for Women and Men

Test	Probably Deficient &/or Pathological Trend	Probably Deficient &/or Pathological Levels	Optimal	Reference Range Young Adults
Thyroid				
TSH	High	≥2.5	1	0.4-2.5 mIU/ml
Free T3	Low	0-2.4	2.5-3.4	1.8-3.7 ng/dl
Free T4	Low	0-1.2	1.3-1.8	0.8-1.8 ng/dl
Reverse T3	High	>30	<25	11-32 ng/dl
Thyroid Antibodies:				
Thyroid Peroxidase TPOAb	High	≥20	0	0-50 U/ml
Thyroglobulin TRAb	High	≥20	0	0-50 U/ml
Thyrotropin receptor TgAb	High	≥5	0	0-10 U/ml
Pregnenolone	Low	<50	50-200	10-200 ng/dl
Aldosterone	Low	0-10	>15	4-30 ng/dl
Sodium	Low	0-138	141	136-145 mmol/l
Potassium	High	>4.8	4.3	3.5-5.1 mmol/l
Cortisol				
a.m.	Low	0-13	18 to 25	10-30 ng/ml
p.m.	Low	0-7	10 to 12	2-20 ng/ml
ACTH	Low/High	<25 or >70	45	20-80 mg/l
Glucose (fasting)	Low/High	<80 or >95	80-95	60-110 mg/dl
Insulin (fasting)	Low/High	<3 or >10	4-9	4-25 uIU/ml
Hb A1c	High	>6	4.5-6.0	4-7%
Vitamin D3 (25-OH)	Low	<30	50-60	20-100 ng/ml
Ferritin	Low	<70	70-90	10-105 ng/ml
Magnesium (RBC)	Low	<4	5.0-6.4	4.0-6.4 mg/dl

*Selected blood test data adapted with approval from The Hormone Handbook, by Thierry Hertoghe, M.D., which can be ordered at www.imbooks.info.

Appendix B

Doctor Referrals

The following are resources for locating physicians who specialize in hormone testing and bio-identical hormone replacement. The first five referral sources include physician locator options on their websites. You simply enter your zip code or city and doctors in your area are identified.

- **American College for Advancement in Medicine (ACAM)**
  24411 Ridge Route, Ste. 115
  Laguna Hills, CA 92653
  Phone: (949) 309-3520
  Website: http://www.acamnet.org

- **American Academy of Anti-Aging Medicine (A4M)**
  1510 W. Montana Street
  Chicago, IL 60614
  Phone: (773) 528-1000
  Website: http://www.worldhealth.net/ (Click on "Directory.")

- **American Holistic Medical Association**
  12101 Menaul Boulevard, NE, Suite C
  Albuquerque, NM 87112
  Phone: 505-292-7788
  Website: http://www.holisticmedicine.org/

- **Health Professionals Directory**
  Website: http://www.healthprofs.com/cam/

- **Doctors who prescribe Armour Thyroid referral site**
  http://thyroid-info.com/topdrs/armour.htm

- **International Academy of Compounding Pharmacists (IACP)**
  Compounding pharmacies make individualized bio-identical hormones and the staff generally knows which local doctors prescribe them. For a referral in your area contact IACP at (800) 927-4227 or at www.iacprx.org.

- **Phone book**
  Look in the yellow pages under "physicians". Hormone specialists often advertise themselves as holistic physicians.

- **The International Hormone Society**
  7 Avenue Van Bever, 1180 Brussels, Belgium
  Website: www.intlhormonesociety.org

- **The World Society of Anti-Aging Medicine**
  Website: www.wosaam.org

References

Chapter I Finding the MS Solution: My Journey with MS

[1] Lorand, A. 1915. *Old Age Deferred*. Philadelphia: F.A. Davis.
[2] DeGroot, L., P. Larsen, and G. Hennemann, 1996. *The Thyroid and Its Diseases*. New York: Churchill Livingstone.

Chapter II Multiple Sclerosis: An Inflammatory Process

[1] Health-Cares. 2005. What types of multiple sclerosis are there? http://neurology.health-cares.net/multiple-sclerosis-types.php.
[2] Lubetzki, C., C. Demerens, P. Anglade, H. Villarroya, A. Frankfurter, V.M. Lee, and B. Zalc. 1993. Even in culture, oligodendrocytes myelinate solely axons. *Proceedings of the National Academy of Sciences* 90:6820–6824.
[3] Garcia-Segura, L.M., and M.M. McCarthy. 2003. Minireview: role of glia in neuroendocrine function. *Endocrinology* 145(3):1082–1086.
[4] Alam, M., and W.J. Schmidt. 2004. Mitochondrial complex I inhibition depletes plasma testosterone in the rotenone model of Parkinson's disease. *Physiology & Behavior* 83:395–400.
[5] Ragonese, P., M. D'Amelio, G. Salemi, P. Aridon, M. Gammino, A. Epifanio, L. Morgante, and G. Savettieri. 2004. Risk of Parkinson's disease in women: effect of reproductive characteristics. *Neurology* 62:2010–2014.
[6] Chen, H., S.M. Zhang, M.A. Hernana, M.A. Schwarzschild, W.C. Willett, G.A. Colditz, F.E. Speizer, and A. Ascherio. 2003. Nonsteroidal anti-inflammatory drugs and the risk of Parkinson's disease. *Archives of Neurology* 60:1059–1064.
[7] Chung, H.Y., H.J. Kim, K.W. Kim, J.S. Choi, and B.P. Yu. 2003. Molecular inflammation hypothesis of aging based on the anti-aging mechanism of calorie restriction. *Microscopy Research and Technique* 59:264–272.
[8] Loesche, W.J. 1994. Periodontal disease as a risk factor for heart disease. *Compendium* 15(8):976, 978–982, 985–986.

Chapter III Sex Hormones and MS *for Women*

[1] Health-Cares. 2005. What types of multiple sclerosis are there? http://neurology.health-cares.net/multiple-sclerosis-types.php.
[2] Jasienska, G., A. Ziomkiewicz, P.T. Ellison, S.F. Lipson, and I. Thrune. 2004. Large breasts and narrow waists indicate high reproductive potential in women. *Proceedings. Biological Sciences / The Royal Society* 271:1213–1217.

[3] Tomassini, V., E. Onesti, C. Mainero, E. Giugni, A. Paolillo, M. Salvetti, F. Nicoletti, and C. Pozzilli. 2005. Sex hormones modulate brain damage in multiple sclerosis: MRI evidence. *Journal of Neurology, Neurosurgery, and Psychiatry* 76:272–275.

[4] Polanczyk, M. 2003. The protective effect of 17ß-estradiol on experimental autoimmune encephalomyelitis is mediated through estrogen receptor. *American Journal of Pathology* 63:1599–1605.

[5] Cutolo, M., B. Seriolo, B. Villagio, C. Pizzorni, C. Craviotto, and A. Sulli. 2002. Androgens and estrogens modulate the immune and inflammatory responses in rheumatoid arthritis. *Annals of the New York Academy of Sciences* 966(1):131–142.

[6] Turgeon, J.L., M.C. Carr, P.M. Maki, M.E. Mendelsohn, and P.M. Wise. 2006. Complex actions of sex steroids in adipose tissue, the cardiovascular system, and brain: insights from basic science and clinical studies. *Endocrine Reviews* 27(6):575.

[7] Nash, J.W., C. Morrison, and W.L. Frankel. 2003. The utility of estrogen receptor and progesterone receptor immunohistochemistry in the distinction of metastatic breast carcinoma from other tumors in the liver. *Archives of Pathology and Laboratory Medicine* 127(12):1591–1595.

[8] Ogueta, S.B., S.D. Schwartz, C.K. Yamashita, and D.B. Farber. 1999. Estrogen receptor in the human eye: influence of gender and age on gene expression. *Investigative Ophthalmology and Visual Science* 40:1906–1911.

[9] Koenig, H.L., M. Schumacher, B. Ferzaz, A.N. Do Thi, A. Ressouches, R. Guennoun, I. Jung-Testas, P. Robel, Y. Akwa, and E.E. Baulieu. 1995. Progesterone synthesis and myelin formation by Schwann cells. *Science* 268:1500–1503.

[10] Schumacher, M., R. Guennoun, A.M. Ghoumari, C. Massaad, F. Robert, M. El-Etr, Y. Akwa, K. Rajkowski, and E.E. Baulieu. 2007. Novel perspectives for progesterone in hormone replacement therapy, with special reference to the nervous system. *Endocrine Reviews* 28(4):387–439.

[11] Peters, A. 1996. Age-related changes in oligodendrocytes in monkey cerebral cortex. *Journal of Comparative Neurology* 371:153–163.

[12] Murphy, S.J., M.T. Littleton-Kearney, and P.D. Hurn. 2002. Progesterone administration during reperfusion, but not preischemia alone, reduces injury in ovariectomized rats. *Journal of Cerebral Blood Flow & Metabolism* 22:1181–1188.

[13] Lutskii, M.A., and I.E. Esaulenko 2007. Oxidant stress in the pathogenesis of multiple sclerosis. *Neuroscience and Behavioral Physiology* 37(3):209–213.

[14] Moorthy, K., D. Sharma, S.F. Basir, and N.Z. Baquer. 2005. Administration of estradiol and progesterone modulate the activities of antioxidant enzyme and aminotransferases in naturally menopausal rats. *Experimental Gerontology* 40:295–302.

[15] Marin-Husstege, M., D. Muggironi, R.P. Raban, P. Skoff, and P. Casaccia-Bonnefil. 2004. Oligodendrocyte progenitor proliferation and maturation is differentially regulated by male and female sex steroid hormones. *Developmental Neuroscience* 26:245–254.

[16] Ghoumari, A.M., C. Ibanez, M. El-Etr, P. Leclerc, B. Eychenne, B.W. O'Malley, E. E. Baulieu, and M. Schumacher. 2003. Progesterone and its metabolites increase myelin basic protein expression in organotypic slice cultures of rat cerebellum. *Journal of Neurochemistry* 86:848–859.

[17] Moggs, J.G. 2005. Molecular responses to xenoestrogens: mechanistic insights into toxicogenomics. *Toxicology* 213(3):177–193.

[18] Tomassini, V., E. Onesti, C. Mainero, E. Giugni, A. Paolillo, M. Salvetti, F. Nicoletti, and C. Pozzilli. 2005. Sex hormones modulate brain damage in multiple sclerosis: MRI evidence. *Journal of Neurology, Neurosurgery, and Psychiatry* 76:272–275.

[19] Hertoghe, T. 2006. *The Hormone Handbook.* Surrey, United Kingdom: International Medical Books.
[20] Lee, J.. 2002. *What Your Doctor May Not Tell You About Breast Cancer.* New York: Warner Books.
[21] Littleton-Kearney, M.T., J.A. Klaus, and P.D. Hurn. 2005. Effects of combined oral conjugated estrogens and medroxyprogesterone acetate on brain infarction size after experimental stroke in rat. *Journal of Cerebral Blood Flow & Metabolism* 25:421–426.
[22] Moyer, D.L., B. de Lignieres, P. Driguez, and J.P. Pez. 1993. Prevention of endometrial hyperplasia by progesterone during long-term estradiol replacement: influence of bleeding pattern and secretory changes. *Fertility and Sterility* 59(5):992–997.
[23] Fanchin, R., D. De Ziegler, C. Bergeron, C. Righini, C. Torrisi, and R. Frydman. 1997. Transvaginal administration of progesterone. *Obstetrics & Gynecology* 90:396–401.
[24] Bebo, B.F., A. Fyfe-Johnson, K. Adlard, A.G. Beam, A.A. Vandenbark, and H. Offner. 2001. Low-dose estrogen therapy ameliorates experimental autoimmune encephalomyelitis in two different inbred mouse strains. *The Journal of Immunology* 166:2080–2089.
[25] Vliet, E.L. 1995. *Screaming to Be Heard: Hormone Connections Women Suspect and Doctors Still Ignore.* New York: M. Evans and Company.
[26] Roungsin, C., and D. Manoch. 2004. Efficacy of oral micronized progesterone when applied via vaginal route. *Journal of the Medical Association of Thailand* 87(5):455–458.
[27] Ibid.

Chapter IV Sex Hormones and MS *for Men*

[1] Medical News Today. 2007. New poll shows men, women incorrectly blame symptoms of low testosterone on normal aging. www.medicalnewstoday.com/articles.
[2] Pugh, P.J., T.H. Jones, and K.S. Channer. 2003. Acute haemodynamic effects of testosterone in men with chronic heart failure. *European Heart Journal* 24:909–915.
[3] Weil, T., and S. Lightman. 1997. The neuroendocrine axis in patients with multiple sclerosis. *Brain* 120:1067–1076.
[4] Zych-Twardowska, E., and A. Wajgt. 1999. Serum prolactin and sex hormone concentrations in patients with multiple sclerosis. *Medical Science Monitor* 5(2):216–220.
[5] Hertoghe, T. 2006. *The Hormone Handbook.* Surrey, U.K.: International Medical Publications.
[6] Koenig, H. L., M. Schumacher, B. Ferzaz, A. N. Do Thi, A. Ressouches, R. Guennoun, I. Jung-Testas, P. Robel, Y. Akwa, and E. E. Baulieu. 1995. Progesterone synthesis and myelin formation by Schwann cells. *Science* 268:1500–1503.
[7] Schumacher, M. R., A. Guennoun, C. Ghoumari, F. Massaad, M. Robert, M. El-Etr, Y. Akwa, K. Rajkowski, and E. Baulieu. 2007. Novel perspectives for progesterone in hormone replacement therapy, with special reference to the nervous system. *Endocrine Reviews* 28 (4):387–439.
[8] Murphy, S.J., M. T. Littleton-Kearney, and P. D. Hurn. 2002. Progesterone administration during reperfusion, but not preischemia alone, reduces injury in ovariectomized rats. *Journal of Cerebral Blood Flow & Metabolism* 22:1181–1188.
[9] Moggs, J.G. 2005. Molecular responses to xenoestrogens: mechanistic insights into toxicogenomics. *Toxicology* 213(3):177–193.
[10] Jain, P., A.W. Rademaker, and K.T. McVary. 2000. Testosterone supplementation for erectile dysfunction: results of a meta-analysis. *Journal of Urology* 164:371–375.

[11] Morgentaler, A., C.O. Bruning, and W.C. DeWolf. 1996. Occult prostate cancer in men with low serum testosterone levels. *JAMA* 276(23):1904–1906.

[12] Hertoghe, T. 2006. *The Hormone Handbook*. Surrey, U.K.: International Medical Publications.

Chapter V Don't Ever Underestimate Your Thyroid

[1] Durrant-Peatfield, B. 2002. *The Great Thyroid Scandal and How to Survive It*. London: Barons Down Publishing.

[2] American Association of Clinical Endocrinologists. 2007. Annual meeting of the American Association of Clinical Endocrinologists. http://www.aace.com/meetings/ams/2007/Endodisfacts.php.

[3] Karni, A.O. 1999. Association of MS with thyroid disorders. *Neurology* 53(4):883–885.

[4] Jellinek, E.H., and R.E. Kelly. 1960. Cerebellar syndrome in myxoedema. *Lancet* 2:225.

[5] Yu, X., R.V.S. Rajala, J.F. McGinnis, F. Li, R.E. Anderson, X. Yan, S. Li, R.V. Elias, R.R. Knapp, X. Zhou, and W. Cao. 2004. Involvement of insulin/phosphoinositide 3-kinase/akt signal pathway in 17 beta-estradiol-mediated neuroprotection. *Journal of Biological Chemistry* 279(13):13086–13094.

[6] Simpson, K. 2007. Brain fog. *Going Bonkers* 1(3):26–27.

[7] DeGroot, Leslie J., G. Hennemann, and P.R. Larsen. 1984. *The Thyroid and Its Diseases*. New York: Churchill Livingston.

[8] Carani, C., A.M. Isidori, A. Granata, E. Carosa, M. Maggi, A. Lenzi, and E.A. Jannini. 2005. Multicenter study on the prevalence of sexual symptoms in male hypo- and hyperthyroid patients. *Journal of Clinical Endocrinology and Metabolism* 90(12):6472–6479.

[9] DeGroot, Leslie J., G. Hennemann, and P.R. Larsen. 1984. *The Thyroid and Its Diseases*. New York: Churchill Livingston.

[10] Simonides, W.S., C. van Hardevald, and P.R. Larsen. 1992. Identification of sequences in the promotor of the fast isoform of sarcoplasmic reticulum Ca-ATPase required for transcriptional activation by thyroid hormone, abstracted. *Thyroid* 2:S-102.

[11] Lanni, A., A. Lombardi, M. Moreno, and F. Goglia. 1998. Effect of 3,5-di-iodo-L-thyronine on the mitochondrial energy-transduction apparatus. *Biochemistry Journal* 330(1):521–526.

[12] Stratmoen, J. 2005. High incidence of hypopituitarism among traumatic brain injury patients. *Neurology Today* 5(3):84–85.

[13] Compston, A. 2000. The genetics of multiple sclerosis. *Journal of Neurovirology* 6(2):S5–S9.

[14] Sajous, C. 1903. *Internal Secretions and Principles of Internal Medicine*. Philadelphia: F.A. Davis.

[15] Wartofsky, L., and K. Burman. 1982. Alterations in thyroid function in patients with systemic illness: the "euthyroid sick syndrome." *Endocrine Review* 3:164–216.

[16] Lowe, J.C. 2000. *The Metabolic Treatment of Fibromyalgia*. Boulder: McDowell Publishing Company.

[17] Ibid.

[18] Sajous, C. 1903. *Internal Secretions and Principles of Internal Medicine*. Philadelphia: F.A. Davis.

[19] Forchheimer, F. 1906. *The Prophylaxis and Treatment of Internal Diseases*. New York: Appleton Press.

[20] De Keyser, J. 1988. Autoimmunity in multiple sclerosis. *Neurology* 38:371–374.

[21] Zych-Twardowska, E., and A. Wajgt. 2001. Blood levels of selected hormones in patients with multiple sclerosis. *Medical Science Monitor* 7(5):1005–1012.

22 Fernandez, M. 2004. Supplementing thyroid hormone may offer new multiple sclerosis treatment. *Proceedings of the National Academy of Sciences* 101:16363–16368.

23 Garcia-Segura, L.M., J.A. Chowen, and F. Naftolin. 1996. Endocrine glia: roles of glial cells in the brain actions of steroid and thyroid hormones and in the regulation of hormone secretion. *Frontiers in Neuroendocrinology* 17:180–211.

24 Stephens, P. 2004. Current issues in thyroid disease management. *Reports During Endocrine Society Audioconference. Endocrine News* 29(2).

25 Hueston, W.J. 2001. Treatment of hypothyroidism. *American Family Physician* 64(10):1717–1724.

26 Miller, K.K. 1998. Central hypothyroidism due to pituitary/hypothalamic dysfunction. *Massachusetts General Hospital Neuroendocrine Clinical Center Bulletin* 4(3).

27 Munteis, E., J. Cano, J.A. Flores, J. Martinez-Rodriguez, J.E. Miret, and M. Roquer. 2007. Relevance of autoimmune thyroid disorders in a Spanish multiple sclerosis cohort. *European Journal of Neurology* 14(9):1048–1052.

Chapter VI It's Not Wise to Ignore Your Adrenals

[1] Van Winsen, L.M.L., D.F.R. Muris, C.H. Polman, C.D. Dijkstra, T.K. van den Berg, and B.M.J. Uitdehaag. 2005. Sensitivity to glucocorticoids is decreased in relapsing remitting multiple sclerosis. *Journal of Clinical Endocrinology & Metabolism* 90(2):734–740.

[2] Michelson, D., L. Stone, E. Galliven, M.A. Magiakou, G.P. Chrousos, E.M. Sternberg, and P.W. Gold. 1994. Multiple sclerosis is associated with alterations in hypo-thalamic-pituitary-adrenal axis function. *Journal of Clinical Endocrinology & Metabolism* 79:848–853.Erkut, Z.A., E. Endert, I. Huitinga, and D.F. Swaab. 2002. Cortisol is increased in postmortem cerebrospinal fluid of multiple sclerosis patients: relationship with cytokines and sepsis. *Journal of Clinical Endocrinology & Metabolism* 84:4149–4154.

[3] Then Bergh, T.F., T. Kumpfel, A. Grasser, R. Rupprecht, F. Holsboer, and C. Trenkwalder. 2001. Combined treatment with corticosteroids and moclobemide favors normalization of hypothalamo-pituitary-adrenal axis dysregulation in relapsing-remitting multiple sclerosis: a randomized, double blind trial. *Journal of Clinical Endocrinology & Metabolism* 86:1610–1615.

[4] Michelson, D., L. Stone, E. Galliven, M.A. Magiakou, G.P. Chrousos, E.M. Sternberg, and P.W. Gold. 1994. Multiple sclerosis is associated with alterations in hypothalamic-pituitary-adrenal axis function. *Journal of Clinical Endocrinology & Metabolism* 79:848–853.

[5] Laughlin, G.A., and E. Barret-Connor. 2000. Sexual dimorphism in the influence of advanced aging on adrenal hormone levels: the Rancho Bernardo Study. *Journal of Clinical Endocrinology* 85(10):3561–3568.

[6] Jiang, S., J. Lee, Z. Zhang, P. Inserra, D. Solkoff, and R.R. Watson. 1998. Dehydroepiandrosterone synergizes with antioxidant supplements for immune restoration in old as well as retrovirus-infected mice. *Journal of Nutritional Biochemistry* 9:362.

[7] Vollenhoven, R.F.V., E.G. Engleman, and J.L. McGuire. 1994. An open study of dehydro-epiandrosterone in systemic lupus erythematosus. *Arthritis Rheumatism* 37:1305.

[8] Hertoghe, T. 2006. *The Hormone Handbook*. Surrey, U.K.: International Medical Books.

Chapter VII And Let's Not Forget…the Other Hormones

[1] Ye, P., J. Carson, and A.J. D'Ercole. 1995. In vivo actions of insulin-like growth factor-l (IGF-1) on brain myelination: studies of IGF-1 and IGF binding protein-l (IGF-BP-1) transgenic mice. *The Journal of Neuroscience* 75(11):7344–7356.

[2] Ibid.

[3] Adamopoulos, S., J.T. Parissis, M. Georgiadis, D. Karatzas, J. Paraskevaidis, C. Kroupis, G. Karavolias, K. Koniavitou, and D.T. Kremastinos. 2002. Growth hormone administration reduces circulating proinflammatory cytokines and soluble Fas/soluble Fas ligand system in patients with chronic heart failure secondary to idiopathic dilated cardiomyopathy. *American Heart Journal* 144:359–364.

[4] Chan, J.M., M.J. Stampfer, E. Giovannucci, P.H. Gann, J. Ma, P. Wilkinson, C.H. Hennekens, and M. Pollak. 1998. Plasma insulin-like growth factor-1 and prostate cancer risk: a prospective study. *Science* 279:563–566.

[5] Hertoghe, T. 2006. *The Hormone Handbook*. Surrey, U.K.: International Medical Publications.

[6] Van den Berghe, G. 2000. Novel insights into the neuroendocrinology of critical illness. *European Journal of Endocrinology* 143:1–13.

[7] Harada, J.M., Y. Yamaguchi, N. Shida, and I. Goto. 1991. Hyperprolactinemia in multiple sclerosis. *Journal of the Neurological Sciences* 102:61–66.

[8] Yu-Lee, L. 2002. Prolactin modulation of immune and inflammatory responses. *Recent Progress in Hormone Research* 57:435–455.

[9] Straub, R.H., J. Georgi, K. Helmke, P. Vaith, and B. Lang. 2002. In polymyalgia rheumatica serum prolactin is positively correlated with the number of typical symptoms but not with typical inflammatory markers. *Rheumatology* 41:423–429.

[10] Ibid.

[11] Hertoghe, T. 2006. *The Hormone Handbook*. Surrey, U.K.: International Medical Publications.

[12] Guth, L., Z. Zhang, and E. Roberts. 1994. Key role for pregnenolone in combination therapy that promotes recovery after spinal cord injury. *Proceedings of the National Academy of Sciences* 91(25):12308–12312.

[13] Holick, M.F. 2004. Sunlight and vitamin D for bone health and prevention of autoimmune diseases, cancers, and cardiovascular disease. *American Journal of Clinical Nutrition* 80:1678S–1688S.

[14] Mathieu, C., M. Waer, J. Laureys, O. Rutgeerts, and R. Bouillon. 1994. Prevention of autoimmune diabetes in NOD mice by 1,25 dihydroxyvitamin D3. *Diabetologia* 37:552–558.

[15] Hernan, M.A., M.J. Olek, and A. Ascherio. Geographic variation of MS incidence in two prospective studies of US women. *Neurology* 51:1711–1718.

[16] Armas, L.G., B.W. Hollis, and R.P. Heaney. 2004. Vitamin D2 is much less effective than vitamin D3 in humans. *The Journal of Clinical Endocrinology & Metabolism* 89(11):5387-5391.

[17] Gorham, E.D., C.F. Garland, F.C. Garland, S.B. Mohr, W.B. Grant, M. Lipkin, H.L. Newmark, E. Giovannucci, M.F. Holick, and M. Wei. 2007. Optimal vitamin D status for colorectal cancer prevention: a quantitative meta analysis. *American Journal of Preventative Medicine* 32(3):210–216.

[18] Sandyk, R., and G.I. Awerbuch. 1993. Multiple sclerosis: the role of the pineal gland in its timing of onset and risk of psychiatric illness. *International Journal of Neuroscience* 72(1–2):95–106.

[19] Sandyk R., and G.I. Awerbuch. 1994. Relationship of nocturnal melatonin levels to duration and course of multiple sclerosis. *International Journal of Neuroscience* 75:229–237.

[20] Simon, D., et al. 1992. Interrelation between plasma testosterone and plasma insulin in healthy adult men: the Telecom Study. *Diabetologia* 35(2):173–177.

[21] Watson, G.S., and S. Craft. 2006. Insulin resistance, inflammation, and cognition in Alzheimer's disease: lessons for multiple sclerosis. *Journal of Neurological Sciences* 245(1-2):21–33.

[22] Dorman, J.S., A.R. Steenkiste, J.P. Burke, and M. Songini. 2003. Type 1 diabetes and multiple sclerosis: together at last. *Diabetes Care* 26:3192–3193.

[23] Castro, J.H., S.M. Genuth, and L. Klein. 1975. Comparative response to parathyroid hormone in hyperthyroidism and hypothyroidism. *Metabolism* 4(7):839–848.

Chapter VIII What Else Does Your Body Need?

[1] U.S. News & World Report. 2005. http://health.usnews.com/usnews/health/articles/050328/28sugar.b.htm

[2] United States Department of Agriculture. 2002. Agriculture Fact Book. http://www.usda.gov/factbook/chapter2.htm. Accessed October 10, 2007.

[3] Marshall, B.H. 1991. Lipids and neurological diseases. *Medical Hypotheses* 34(3):272–274.

[4] Di Biase, A., and S. Salvati. 1997. Exogenous lipids in myelination and myelination. *Kaohsiung Journal of Medical Science* 13(1):19–29.

[5] Goldberg, R.J., and J. Katz. 2007. A meta-analysis of the analgesic effects of omega-3 polyunsaturated fatty acid supplementation for inflammatory joint pain. *Pain* 129(1-2):210–223.

[6] Lu, L.J., K.E. Anderson, J.J. Grady, F. Kohen, and M. Nagamani. 2000. Decreased ovarian hormones during a soya diet: Implications for breast cancer prevention. *Cancer Research* 60(15):4112–21.

[7] Bottiglieri, T. 1996. Folate, vitamin B12, and neuropsychiatric disorders. *Nutritional Review* 54(12):382–90.

[8] Baig S.M., and G. Ali Qureshi. 1995. Homocysteine and vitamin B12 in multiple sclerosis. *Biogenic Amines* 11(6):479–485.

[9] Yasui, M., and K. Ota. 1992. Experimental and clinical studies on dysregulation of magnesium metabolism and the aetiopathogenesis of multiple sclerosis. *Magnesium Research* 5(4):295–302.

[10] Goldberg, P., M.C. Fleming, and E.H. Picard. 1986. Multiple sclerosis: decreased relapse rate through dietary supplementation with calcium, magnesium and vitamin D. *Medical Hypotheses* 21(2):193–200.

[11] Yasui, M., and K. Ota. 1992. Experimental and clinical studies on dysregulation of magnesium metabolism and the aetiopathogenesis of multiple sclerosis. *Magnesium Research* 5(4):295–302.

[12] Yasui, M., Y. Yase, K. Ando, K. Adachi, M. Mukoyama, and K. Ohsugi. 1990. Magnesium concentration in brains from multiple sclerosis patients. *Acta Neurologica Scandinavica* 81(3):197–200.

[13] Rossier, P. 2000. Clinical correspondence: the effect of magnesium oral therapy on spasticity in a patient with multiple sclerosis. *European Journal of Neurology* 7(6):741–4.

[14] Johnson, S. 2000. The possible role of gradual accumulation of copper, cadmium, lead and iron and gradual depletion of zinc, magnesium, selenium, vitamins B2, B6, D, and E and essential fatty acids in multiple sclerosis. *Medical Hypotheses* 55(3):239–241.

Index

A
"ABC" drugs, 131
abdominal pain, 128
acetaminophen, 71
acetyl-L-carnitine, 179
acne, 138
ACTH, 134–35, 137, 189
adrenals. *See also* cortisol; DHEA (dehydroepiandrosterone)
    adrenal dysfunction, 125–26
    adrenal fatigue, 15, 122–23, 128
    adrenal hormones, 121, 129, 135, 145–46
    effects of compromised function, 123, 139, 173
    endocrine interrelationships, 14–15, 48, 74, 110–11, 127–28
    evaluating function, 15, 134–35
    feedback loop, 123
    functions, 23, 121
    and thyroid supplementation, 117–18, 129
    treating dysfunction, 117, 136–38, 178
advanced glycation endproducts (AGEs), 32
age
    effect on endocrine function, 24
    and hormone production, 36, 49, 63, 124
    and MS, 24, 35, 36, 44
    neurologic effects, 33, 43
aging, accelerated, 128
AIDS, 144
alcohol
    effects on liver metabolism, 69
    endocrine system effects, 100, 113, 127, 128, 167
    and excess estrogen, 70
    and insulin, 169
    thyroid and alcoholism, 99
aldosterone, 135, 145, 189
allergies, 25, 128, 172–73
Alora, 55
alpha-linolenic fatty acid. *See* omega-3 fatty acids
ALS (Lou Gherig's Disease), 7
Alzheimer's disease, 40, 150
amino acids, 10, 11, 12, 113, 159–60, 179
anastrozole (Arimidex), 71
andropause, 64–65, 92
anemia, 92
anger, 138
angina, 73
anticonvulsant drugs, 700
antidepressants, 47, 71, 75
antifungal drugs, 70
anti-inflammatory agents
    drugs, 21, 28
    hormones, 20–21, 23, 27, 66–67, 68, 129
    statin drugs, 21, 70, 71, 146
    supplements, 179
antioxidants, 176–77
antipsychotic drugs, 70
anti-thyroid antibodies, 109, 112, 189
anxiety, 25, 92, 127, 128
appetite, 92, 127
arachidonic acid, 32
arginine, 11
Arimidex (anastrozole), 71
Armour thyroid, 114–15, 116
aromatase, 68, 69, 70
arthralgia. *See* pain
arthritis, 144, 146–47, 175
artificial sweeteners, 169
Aspartame, 169
aspirin, 71
asthma, 92, 128
astrocytes, 27
attention deficit/hyperactivity disorder (ADHD), 92

autoimmunity
    and adrenal function, 123, 127, 139
    demyelination, 19
    hormone effects, 38, 98, 144, 146–48
    lupus, 144
    T1 pro-inflammatory condition, 27
    triggers, 123, 173
Avonex, 19, 131, 165
axons, 27–28, 29

B

back pain, 5, 8, 128
balance problems, 5, 12, 24, 29, 44, 89
benign prostate hypertrophy, 79, 83
betaine hydrochloride, 173, 180
Betaseron, 19, 131
beta-sitosterol, 70
BHA and BHT, 170–71
binding proteins, 67, 70, 81, 142
bio-identical hormones, 13, 50, 61
birth control pills, 51–52
bladder
    and hormones, 12, 24, 41, 74, 88–89
    and MS, 5, 8, 25, 44
blood clots, 73, 74
blood pressure, 52, 92, 127, 128, 175
blood sugar control, 42, 74. *See also* insulin
body shape
    and cortisol, 31–33
    and estrogen, 36, 41, 67–68
    and testosterone, 63
body temperature regulation, 86, 92
bone health, 39, 40, 42, 55, 73, 175. *See also* osteoporosis
bowel problems
    hormonal connections, 12, 24, 88, 127, 128, 162–63, 172–73
    as MS symptom, 5, 25, 44
brain. *See* also lesions of brain and spinal cord
    and diet, 161, 164
    effects of inflammation, 26–28
    gender differences, 91
    and hormone levels, 40, 46, 55, 91, 109, 162–63
    injury, 43, 65, 74

breasts, 36, 92
breathing difficulties, 25, 44, 92
bruising, 92, 127
B vitamin complex, 113, 178

C

cadmium, 100
calcium, 169, 177, 178
calcium channel blockers, 70
calcium regulation, 151, 153
cancer
    colon cancer, 41
    endometrial cancer, 52–53
    prostate, 81, 143
    protection from progesterone, 42, 52–53
    and vitamin D, 146–47
Candida overgrowth, 173
carbohydrates, 150, 156–59, 164
cardiovascular health
    blood pressure, 52, 92, 127, 128, 175
    and hormone levels, 41, 73, 142, 162–63
    hormone replacement therapy (HRT), 51, 52
    hormone supplementation, 55, 58
    vitamin/mineral deficiency, 176–77
carnosine, 179
carpal tunnel syndrome, 88
cataracts, 89
central hypothyroidism, 112
central nervous system (CNS). *See also* demyelination
    dependence on myelin, 28
    estrogen, 28, 36, 38, 40, 54, 91
    and Graves' disease, 106
    inflammation, 26–29
    insulin-like growth factor 1 (IGF-1), 141–42
    magnesium, 177–78
    MS, 29, 109
    nerve transmission, 29
    progesterone, 42–46, 72
    R-lipoic acid, 179
    testosterone, 28, 91
    thyroid function, 16, 85, 109
cervical dysplasia, 92
chlorinated water, 169

ornithine, 11
osteoporosis. *See also* bone health
   exercise, 175
   parathyroid hormone, 151
   sex hormones, 40, 42, 49, 73, 74
   vitamin/mineral deficiency, 176–77
ovaries
   endocrine interrelationships, 48–49, 110
   follicle stimulating hormone, 60
   menopause, 24, 35
   prolactin, 144
   role in controlling inflammation, 23
   soy products, 170
ovulation, 35–37, 39, 46, 48, 57

P

pain, 92. *See also* neuralgia
   hormonal connections, 40, 91, 128, 162–63
   as MS symptom, 5, 44
   therapies, 77
palpitations, 92, 128
pancreas, 150–51, 158, 170
panic attacks, 128
pantothenic acid, 178
parathyroid, 110, 151–53, 178
Parkinson's disease, 28
patch hormones. *See* transdermal hormone delivery
PCBs, 98
perimenopause, 12, 38–39, 44, 48. *See also* menopause
peripheral neuropathy, 3
pesticides, 70, 98
phenylalanine, 11
phytoestrogens, 170. *See also* xenoestrogens
pineal gland, 149, 153
pituitary
   ACTH, 134–35, 137
   adrenal feedback loop, 123
   effect on hormone levels, 46, 75, 141–45
   endocrine interrelationships, 60, 65, 78, 94, 99, 110, 112
   signs of dysfunction, 82
   supporting, 176–77
plaques. *See* lesions of brain and spinal cord

polyunsaturated fats, 160
potassium, 189
precursor hormones, 41, 42, 74, 145–46, 152, 161
prednisolone, 136
prednisone, 136
pregnancy and MS symptoms, 24, 38, 61
pregnenolone, 145–46, 152, 189
premenstrual syndrome, 93
preservatives, 170–71
probiotics, 180
Prochieve, 57
progesterone
   declining, 35, 46–47
   effects on the body, 20–21, 27, 39, 42
   endocrine interrelationships, 110, 144
   and estrogen supplementation, 55, 58
   measuring, 46, 57, 59, 81, 187, 188
   and men's health, 71, 72–77, 79, 83
   neuroprotective effects, 28, 36, 37, 39, 43, 46, 61, 72
   ovulation, 35
   production, 145, 161
   progesterone products, 13, 51, 52
   receptors, 39, 41, 51, 58, 110
   role in MS, 43–46
   and soy products, 170
   supplementation, 52–53, 56–57, 58, 61
progressive supranuclear palsy (PSP), 7
pro-inflammatory substances, 32, 144
prolactin, 47, 75, 144–45, 152, 187, 188
prolonged evoked potentials, 16
Prometrium, 58
prostate
   cancer, 81, 143
   excess estrogen, 68, 70–71, 80
   insulin-like growth factor 1 (IGF-1), 142
   progesterone supplementation, 79
   PSA (prostate-specific antigen), 81, 187
protein, 100, 159–60
Provera, 51
PSA (prostate-specific antigen), 81, 187
psoriasis, 93, 128
psychological problems, 93
PTH (parathyroid hormone), 151–53

R

radiation exposure, 98, 99
radioactive iodine therapy, 105
Rebif, 19
reflux. *See* gastroesophageal reflux
remyelination. *See* myelination/remyelination
reproductive cycle, 35–37
reservatrol, 176–77
restless legs syndrome, 93
reverse T3, 101
rheumatoid arthritis, 38, 138, 144, 146–47, 162–63
R-lipoic acid, 179
Rocaltrol, 148

S

Sajous, Charles, MD, 106
saturated fats, 47, 160
saw palmetto, 70
scar tissue, nerves. *See* lesions of brain and spinal cord
Schwann cells, 27
secondary progressive phase, 24
selenium, 113, 178
sensory function, 29
serotonin, 40
sex hormone binding globulin (SHBG), 67, 70, 81, 83
sex hormones. *See also individual hormones*
 and body shape, 36, 41, 63, 67–68
 defined, 23, 35
 effects of aging, 24, 35, 63–64
 role in fat production, 31
sexual dysfunction
 and endocrine function, 26, 91, 127, 128
 as MS symptom, 25, 76
 neuron damage, 29
 sex hormones, 42, 64, 74
 treatments, 78
sinus infections, 5, 103, 104
skin health, 41, 93, 127, 128
skin patches. *See* transdermal hormone delivery

sleep problems, 92
 and excess cortisol, 127
 and hormone supplementation, 58
 as MS symptom, 5, 25, 44
 related to hormone deficiency, 12, 24, 90
 sex hormones, 36, 40, 42, 74, 90
soft drinks, 169
Solu-Medrol, 122
soy products, 170
spasticity, 178
speech problems, 91
sperm counts, declining, 47, 75
spinal cord lesions. *See* lesions of brain and spinal cord
starvation, 101
statin drugs, 21, 70, 71, 146
steriod therapy, 122, 136
stiffness, 5, 12, 26, 44, 91, 128
stress
 and adrenal function, 125–26, 129, 139
 countering, 175
 effect on vitamin D, 146
 physical effects, 22, 31, 121–22
 thyroid function, 100, 101
stress hormone. *See* cortisol
stroke, 42, 73, 74, 142
sugar, 47, 158–59, 169
sunlight and hormone production, 147, 148
swallowing difficulties, 6, 44, 92
sweating, 92
synthetic hormones, 51–52, 113
Synthroid (levothyroxine), 113

T

T4. *See* thyroid
taurine, 179
T cells, 27, 142
T2 dominance, 27, 66
temperature intolerance, 128
testicles, 23, 65, 110, 144
testosterone
 and adrenal function, 31, 126–27, 138
 and body shape, 63

and central nervous system, 28, 91
and excess estrogen, 67, 68–69, 81
hormone interrelationships, 142, 144, 150
and inflammation, 20–21, 27, 66–67, 68
measuring, 59, 66–67, 80, 83
and MS, 49
production, 48, 63–65, 145, 161
receptors, 28, 63, 72, 110
recommended levels, 78–79, 187, 188
supplementation, 58, 61, 76, 78–79, 81, 83
symptoms of deficiency, 63–65, 89
thyroid function, 72, 110
tetany, 178
TgAb (thyrogolbulin antibodies), 109
thymus gland, 23, 27, 148
thyrogolbulin antibodies (TgAb), 109
thyroid. *See also* hypothyroidism
   anti-thyroid antibodies, 109, 112, 189
   central nervous system effects, 16, 85, 109
   diet, 10, 95, 113, 170
   effect on body systems, 20–21, 23, 69, 85, 86, 119
   endocrine interrelationships, 14–15, 94, 96, 97, 110–11, 151
   hormone types and roles, 13, 94, 95, 101, 104
   hyperthyroidism, 105–6
   measuring function, 13, 96, 111–12, 119, 189
   normalizing, 102
   receptors, 28, 48, 72, 110, 111
   relationship to alcoholism, 99
   and sex hormones, 41, 46, 48, 69, 72, 74, 75
   thyroid dysfunction and MS, 109
   thyroid hormone resistance, 101
   treatment options, 101, 113–18, 129, 137, 178
   T4 to T3 conversion, 100, 102, 114, 170
thyroid stimulating hormone (TSH), 94, 96, 111–12
thyrotropin receptor antibodies (TRAb), 109
tingling, 88, 93, 151, 178
tinnitus, 25, 44, 92
tongue, 91
TPOAb (thyroid peroxidase antibodies), 109
T1 pro-inflammatory condition, 27
TRAb (thyrotropin receptor antibodies), 109

transdermal hormone delivery
   estrogen, 52, 55–56
   testosterone, 58, 78, 83
trans fats, 161–62, 181
trigeminal neuralgia, 131
TSH. *See* thyroid stimulating hormone (TSH)
T4 to T3 conversion. *See* thyroid
tyrosine, 113, 178

U
ulcers, 127
unsaturated fats, 160
urinary tract infections, 93
Urtica dioica, 70

V
vaginal hormone delivery, 53, 57
vision problems
   and endocrine function, 12, 24, 40, 89, 128, 162–63
   estrogen therapy, 89
   as MS symptom, 5, 8, 25
   sensory neuron damage, 29
vitamin D, 146–48
   functions, 27, 147, 151, 152
   preventing MS, 153
   recommended levels, 189
vitamin/mineral deficiency, 176–77
   effect on endocrine system, 47, 75, 100, 102, 151, 152
   neurological dysfunction, 155, 176–77
   sugar, 158
vitamin/mineral supplementation, 155, 176–79, 181
Vivelle-Dot, 55, 56
Vliet, Elizabeth, MD, 55

W
walking, difficulty, 12. *See also* coordination, loss of
waste product buildup, 87, 89
water, drinking, 169, 170
water retention, 42
weakness. *See* muscles

weight, 49. *See also* fat, body
   controlling, 49
   gain, 127, 138
   loss, 31, 128
women's health. *See also* estrogen; progesterone
   effect of aging, 24
   hypothyroidism, 86
   menstrual cycle, 35–37
   recommended hormone levels, 188, 189
   sex hormones and MS, 35–43
   testosterone, 48–49
   yeast infections, 93
Women's Health Initiative (WHI), 50–51

X
xenoestrogens, 47, 70, 75. *See also* phytoestrogens

Y
yeast (Candida) overgrowth, 173

Z
zinc, 69, 70, 75, 113, 177, 178